Personal Development

Book 2

Kenneth Rouse

OXFORD

OXFORD
UNIVERSITY PRESS
AUSTRALIA & NEW ZEALAND

Level 8, 737 Bourke Street, Docklands, Victoria 3008, Australia

Oxford University Press is a department of the University of Oxford. It furthers the University's objective of excellence in research, scholarship, and education by publishing worldwide. Oxford is a registered trademark of Oxford University Press in the UK and in certain other countries.

First published 2005
Reprinted 2006, 2008, 2009, 2012, 2013 (third), 2014 (three times), 2016, 2017 (twice), 2018, 2020, 2023 (twice), 2025

ISBN 978 0 19 555880 7

Typeset by Lynn Twelftree
Printed in China by Golden Cup Printing Co. Ltd.

Oxford University Press Australia & New Zealand is committed to sourcing paper responsibly.

MIX
Paper | Supporting responsible forestry
FSC
www.fsc.org
FSC™ C110497

Acknowledgement
This book was developed with the support of the Australian Government through the Curriculum Reform Implementation Project.

Contents

Grade 7

Grade 8

Secretary's Message

The Upper Primary Personal Development Syllabus is based on the Curriculum Principles of Our Way of Life and Integral Human Development that focus on healthy living, an active lifestyle, pride in our culture, lifestyles and values, the importance of relationships, and living and working together harmoniously. Students will play an informed role in both individual and community actions that will foster physical, social, emotional, mental and spiritual wellbeing.

This syllabus addresses a wide range of personal, social and community health issues such as reproductive health, growth in population, nutrition, physical activity, safety, HIV and AIDS, drugs and alcohol, the abuse of freedom and rights and peer pressure. Topics of this nature are important issues facing our society today.

Consultation and cooperation between school, home and community will ensure the topics are addressed in a way that supports the role of parents and is sensitive to the values, attitudes, beliefs and practices of the community. All students, both female and male, should be encouraged to participate in all activities to enable them to reach their full potential in all aspects of their lives, and to realise the importance of being a respected, responsible citizen.

Student Books 1 and 2, and the accompanying Teacher Resource Book, have been prepared to provide direct support for the achievement of syllabus outcomes. The content is consistent with, and promotes the teaching and learning models of, the syllabus and the related Department of Education Teachers Guide. These resources encompass a range of material including student activities, advice to teachers, assessment ideas, homework activities, project activities, reference information and a glossary of terms. They are intended to facilitate flexible learning activities for teachers and students, and may be modified and amended to suit local circumstances.

I commend and approve these materials for use in all Upper Primary schools throughout Papua New Guinea.

Peter M. Baki

PETER M BAKI CBE
Secretary for Education

1 GRADE 7 Relationships

Chapter Summary

In this chapter you will have an opportunity to:

- ✔ Find out what is meant by different types of family and the roles that they play
- ✔ Find out about the way that people behave in different groups
- ✔ Describe the differences and similarities between different people
- ✔ Describe how the roles that people play affect relationships
- ✔ Find out how to maintain effective relationships

Syllabus references

Strand: Relationships
Sub-strand: Interactions in relationships and groups

Outcomes:

7.1.1 Describe different types of families and the roles of family members

7.1.2 Develop codes of behaviour appropriate to different relationships and groups

7.1.3 Describe differences between people and their similarities

7.1.4 Outline how taking on different roles affects relationships, attitudes and behaviour

7.1.5 Demonstrate skills needed to maintain effective relationships

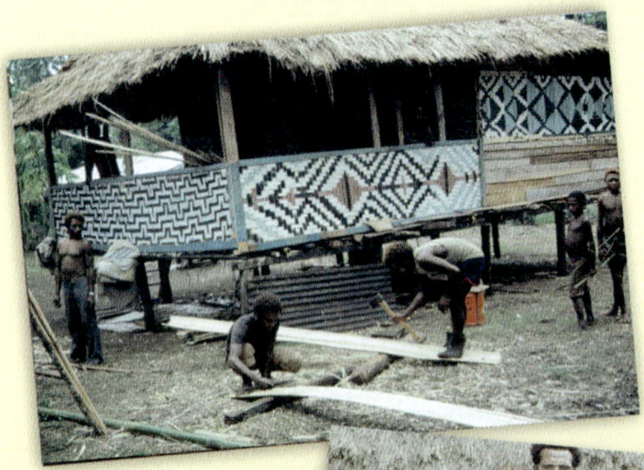

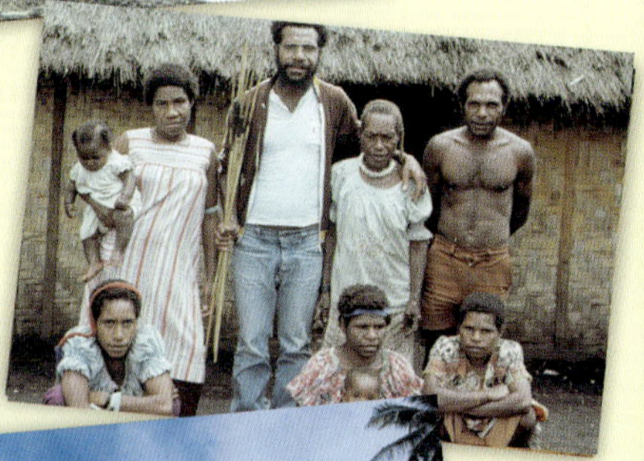

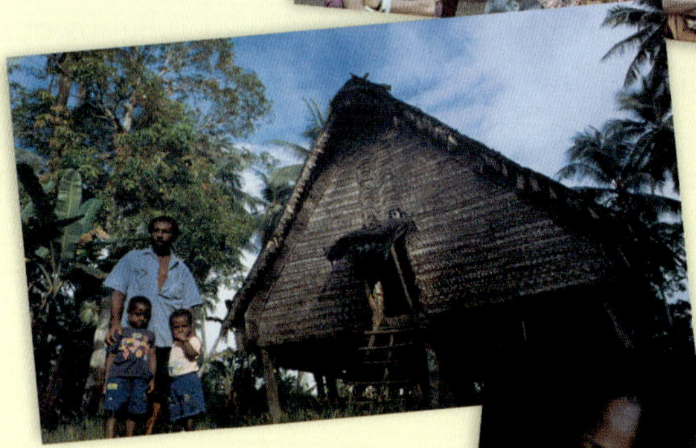

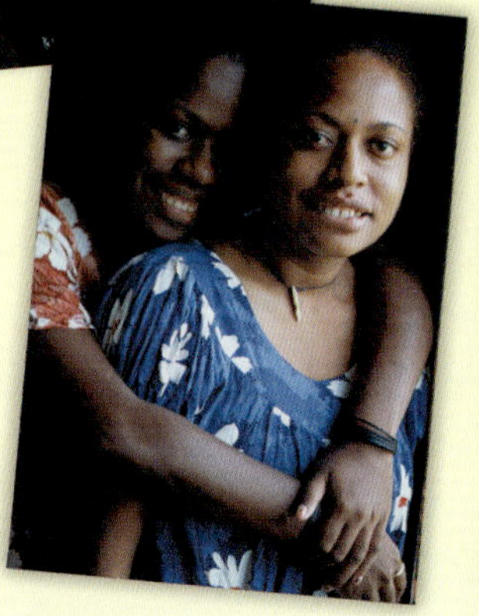

Interaction in relationships and groups

TYPES OF FAMILIES

Key facts

- There are a number of different types of families and people play different roles in each family.
- There is an accepted code of behaviour for each relationship and group.
- People can be described by their similarities to and differences from each other.
- When we take on a particular role, this affects our relationships, attitude and behaviour.
- Skills are needed to maintain effective relationships.

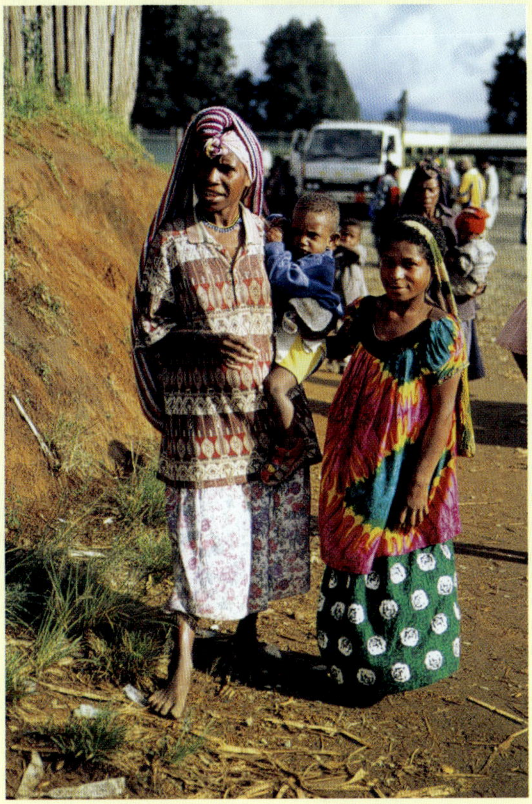

We are all members of a family although there are many different types of families. Families can be different in the same country and can also be different in other countries in the world. The main types of family are the following:

- **Extended family** Children live with their parents, grandparents and possibly other relatives too, or other relatives live nearby. This type of family is found in many parts of Papua New Guinea.
- **Nuclear family** Children live with their parents, and possibly with another relative, although most relatives may be living a long way away.

- **Single parent family** When one parent dies, or when a couple get divorced, then the children may be brought up in a family where there is only one parent. This is called a single parent family.
- **Polygamy** When a man has more than one wife, or a woman has more than one husband, this is called polygamy. Polygamy is found in some parts of Papua New Guinea.
- **Polyandry** When a woman has more than one husband, this is called polyandry. The woman may have children who have different fathers. Polyandry is one kind of polygamy.
- **Polygyny** When a man has more than one wife, this is called polygyny. The man may have children with each of his wives. Each wife may live in her own house away from the other wives to prevent arguments. Polygyny is one kind of polygamy.
- **De facto** A man and woman living together, although they are not married. There may be children in this family, or the couple may not have children.
- **Blended family** After someone dies or after a couple get divorced, a man or woman might get married again. When both husband and wife have children from the previous marriage then they all live together. This type of family is becoming more common in developed countries.

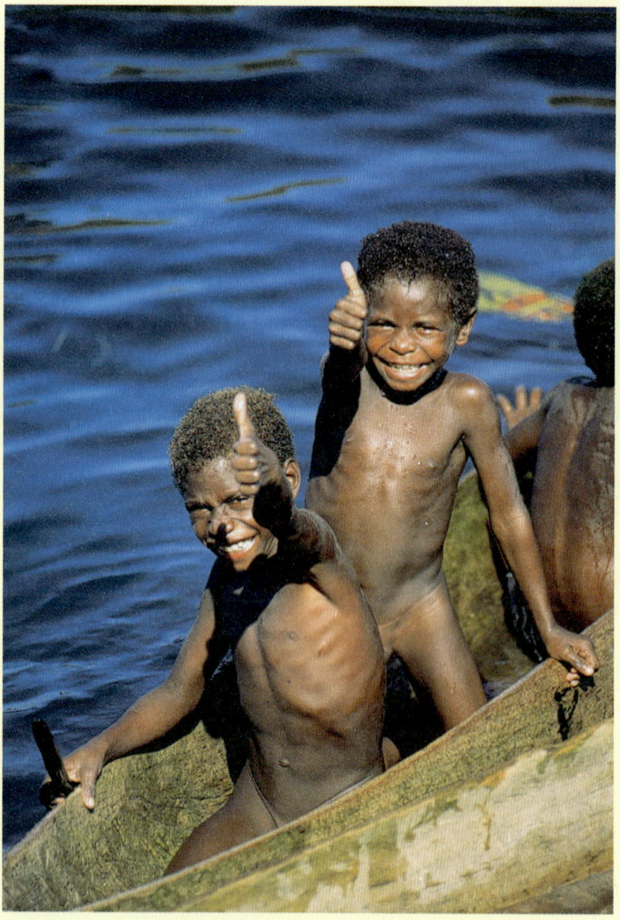

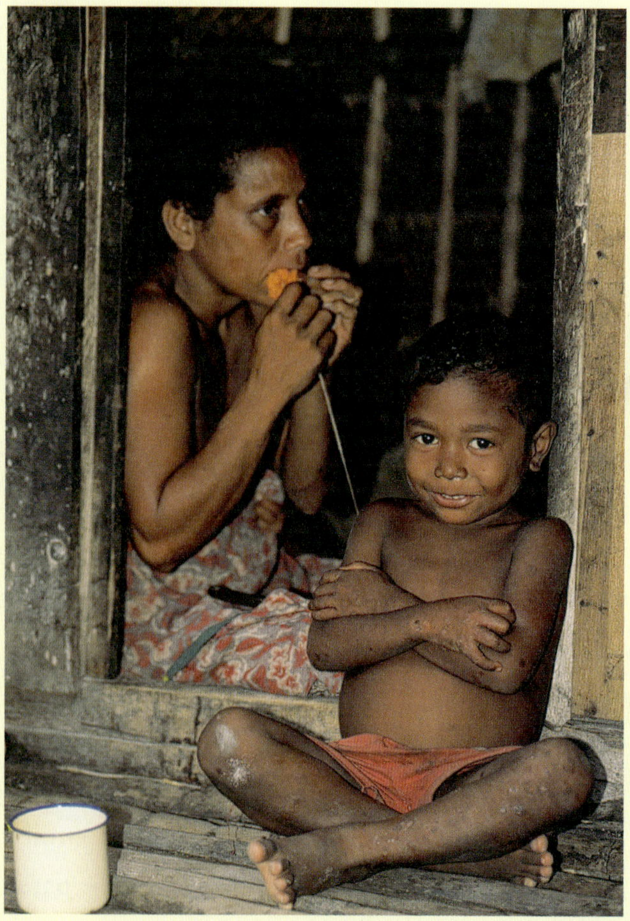

ROLES OF DIFFERENT TYPES OF FAMILY ML

Because families are different they may meet the needs of different family members in different ways. For example, in an extended family, people share the different roles and responsibilities. There are many adults to share the work, take care of children and look after old people. The extended family is able to look after members of the family, especially when they need help—like paying school fees, for example, or when people are sick.

In a nuclear family, children may not know some of their relatives very well and may not be able to learn from them.

Although families may be different, they all share some characteristics in common. For example:

- Families help meet basic human needs such as housing, food and clothing.
- Families provide respect, comfort, love and security.
- Families provide support for healthy and happy living.

For you to try

- Describe the different kinds of families that are found in your area.
- Copy and complete the following table:

Type of family	Advantages	Disadvantages
Extended family		
Nuclear family		

- Choose some different kinds of families and compare the similarities and differences.
- Make a list of the responsibilities of people in different relationships.
- Imagine that you come from a polygamous family where your father has more than one wife or your mother has more than one husband. Describe what you think your life would be like. If you come from a polygamous family, describe what you think your life would be like if you came from a different kind of family.

CODES OF BEHAVIOUR FOR DIFFERENT RELATIONSHIPS

We all have relationships with the people in our family and with people outside our family. We usually have a special relationship with our own family, but we can also learn to feel very close to people outside the family. We are usually expected to behave in certain ways with people inside our family, which may be different from the ways that we behave with people from outside. These different ways that we behave in relationships are sometimes called **codes of behaviour**.

In our relationships with others we need to learn to do the following things:

- make good decisions about the things that we do in our lives
- develop respect for other people
- feel positive about ourselves and about other people
- recognise the needs of other people
- listen to the opinions of other people
- develop positive values like being trustworthy, helpful and sharing
- be assertive. This means that we need to be confident to say what we think.

DEALING WITH PROBLEMS

Most people have problems with other people at some time. The problems or disagreements that we have with other people are called **conflict**. Some of these problems may be caused by the different **expectations** that people have. Other people may want us to do certain things or to behave in certain ways and we may not always feel like doing what they want. For example, children in a family are expected to listen carefully to what the adults say and to show respect. When children do not listen to and obey their parents then there is conflict between the parents and children and the parents may punish the children.

Most parents usually want their children to do the following:

- behave in ways that are acceptable to the family or group
- know what behaviour is expected at different times and places
- understand the reasons why we behave in certain ways
- learn to make good decisions for themselves as they get older

In order to deal with the problems that we have with other people we all need to be able to

- tell others how we are feeling
- give our point of view without getting angry or fighting
- learn what to do when other people get angry

For you to try

- List some of the reasons why you feel positive about yourself and other people.
- List some of the needs of other people.
- List some more positive values of people, like being trustworthy, helpful and sharing.
- Describe some examples of behaviour that is acceptable to your family or a group that you know. Why is this behaviour acceptable? What happens to people who behave well?
- Describe some examples of behaviour that is unacceptable to your family or a group that you know. Why is this behaviour unacceptable? What happens to people who behave badly?

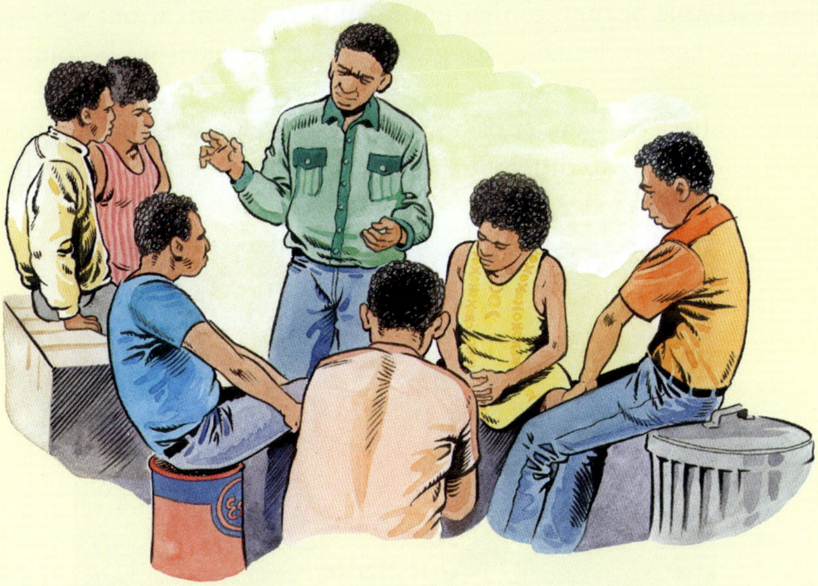

For you to try

- Make a list of the different types of relationship that you have with people at home, in the community and at school. Choose one of those relationships and describe the ways that you can use to develop that relationship.
- With a group of other students, discuss the behaviour that you think helps to make a good relationship between people. Make a list of all the behaviour that you think of.
- Write a story about two people who had a good relationship. Describe how the relationship began and how they kept the relationship going.
- Think about a good friendship or relationship that you have now, or have had in the past. Why was it a good? How did the relationship make you feel?

Cultural and personal identity

DIFFERENCES AND SIMILARITIES BETWEEN PEOPLE

There are many differences and similarities between people. These differences and similarities mean that we are a member of some groups, but not a member of others. For example, boys and men belong to a group that we call 'male'. Girls and women belong to a group which we call 'female'. After being born as a male or female we learn from our community how to become girls and boys, men and women. This is called **gender**. Gender includes all the characteristics of belonging to the male or female sex, as well as the characteristics, behaviour and attitudes of being male or female that come from the community in which we grow up. We will always belong to the same gender and cannot choose another group.

Another group that you belong to is your age group. For example, students in Grade 7 are all about fourteen years old, so everyone belongs to that group and shares similarities with other members of the group. Of course, no one stays in the same age group. As we get older we become a member of a different age group.

Although we cannot choose our gender or our age, we can choose to belong to other groups. For example, we can choose to belong to different sports groups, or to a particular religion or church group.

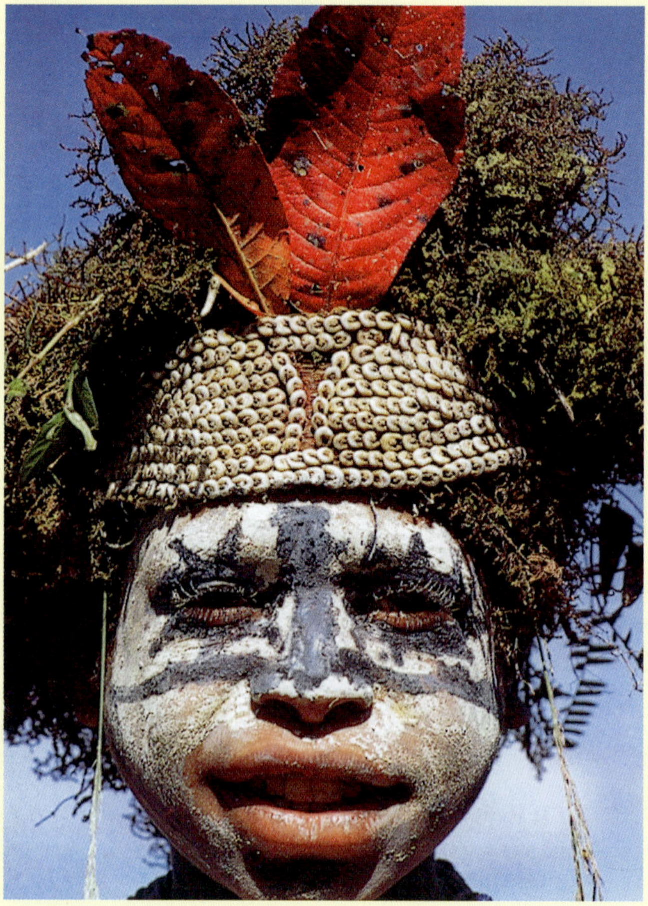

People who belong to the same group usually share some characteristics in common. For example:

- They often have the same interests.
- They often carry out the same activities.
- They often share the same values.
- They often wear similar dress or have similar appearance.
- They sometimes have the same diet.

We learn to be a member of a group and to share the same values in a number of different ways:

- by copying
- by being told by others and by asking questions
- by following tradition
- by making use of opportunities

Identity and respect

Each of us has an **identity** that is affected by the people around us and by the groups to which we belong. The type of food that we eat, the language that we speak and the way that we dress all affect our identity.

We expect others to respect us as individuals and to respect the group to which we belong. In the same way, we also need to respect other individuals and groups who are different to us.

The way that we dress is part of our cultural identity.

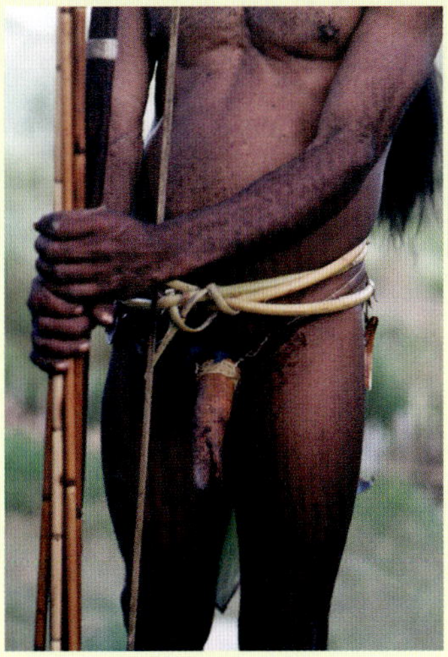

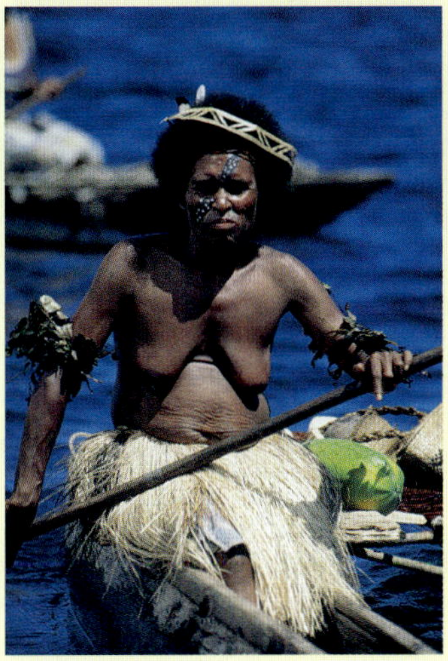

For you to try

- Choose some different cultural groups. Make a list of their similarities and differences.
- Think about a group that is different from you, with a different language and culture, or a different religion. Describe how you show respect for that group and your reasons for behaving in this way.

Changing roles and responsibilities

ROLES AND THE EFFECTS ON RELATIONSHIPS, ATTITUDES AND BEHAVIOUR

At different times we all have to take on different roles in the groups that we belong to. For example, we might be a team leader, a team member, or even a coach. Some people like to be leaders and some do not. Some people like to be a team member first and to get some practice or experience before they feel comfortable being a team leader. If everyone has a turn at being the leader, then it helps us all to understand what it is like to be in the position of being a leader.

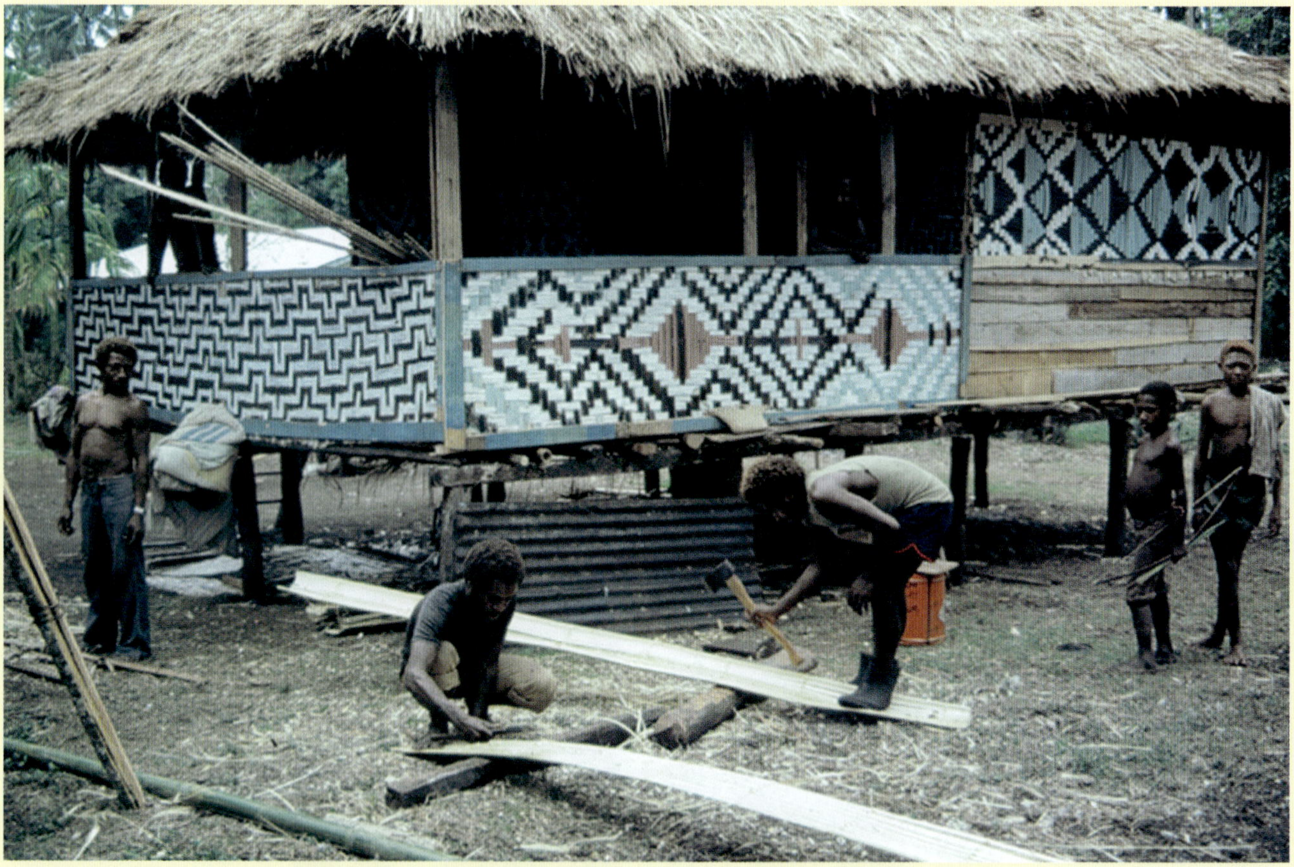

When people work together in a group, they sometimes agree on a set of ground rules to help the group work well together. Some examples of ground rules are:

- Speak kindly and clearly, openly and honestly.
- Discuss common problems and find solutions together.

- Help each other when there is work to be done.
- Be patient with each other.
- Be tolerant with each other, especially when mistakes are made.
- Be trustworthy and reliable.

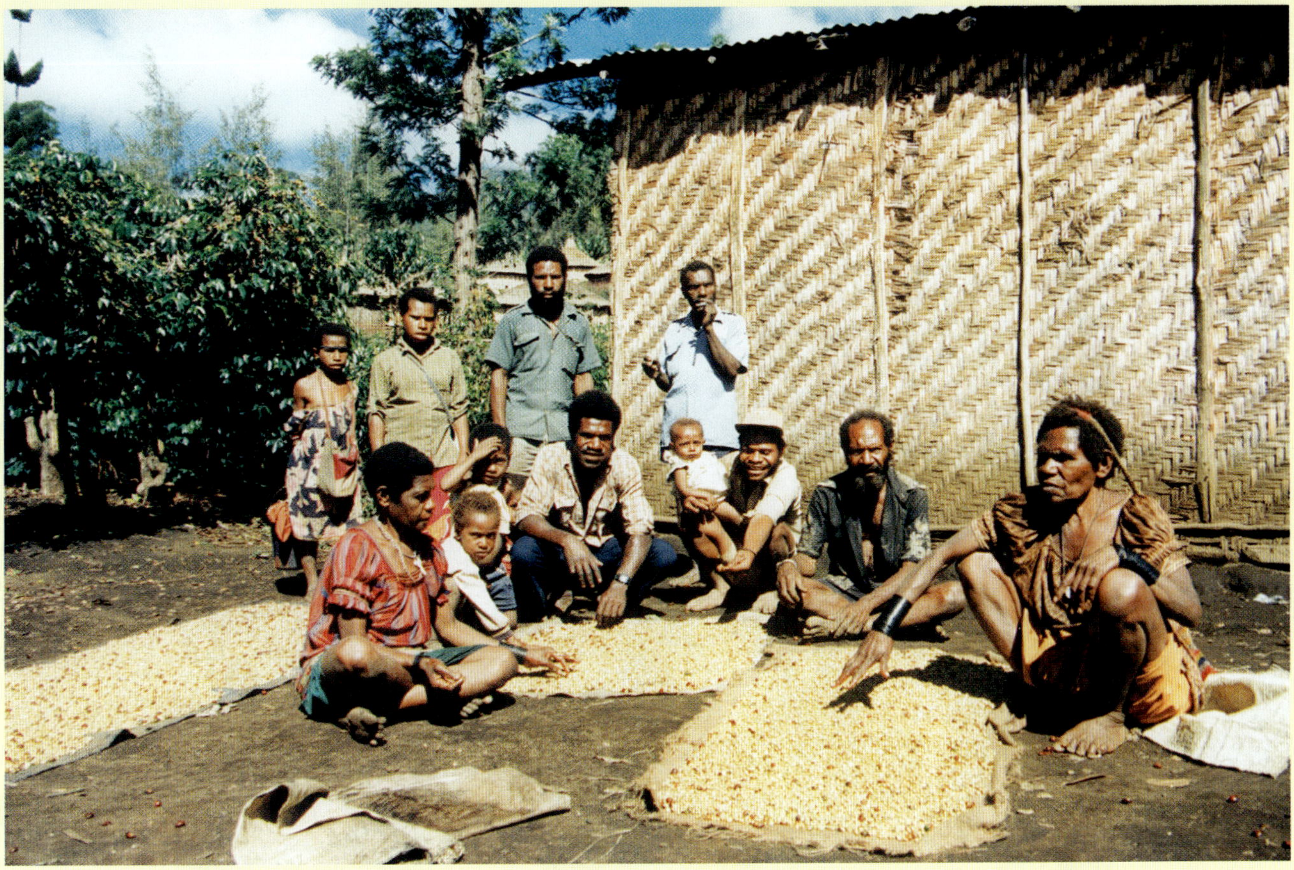

For you to try

- Choose a group and an activity for that group. List the roles and responsibilities that need to be carried out by that group. Describe the responsibilities that you feel you can carry out in the group.
- Describe how taking on responsibilities in a group can affect the relationships, attitudes and behaviour of members of the group.

Managing relationships

HOW TO MAINTAIN EFFECTIVE RELATIONSHIPS

In order to live and work happily with other people, there are a number of things that we can do to make our relationships work well:

- Listen carefully to others.
- Respect other people and what they say.
- Speak kindly and firmly but without being aggressive.
- Be positive in your attitudes to yourself and to other people.
- Think positively about the ways to solve problems.
- Try to find peaceful solutions.
- Let other people know what is happening, when they need to know.

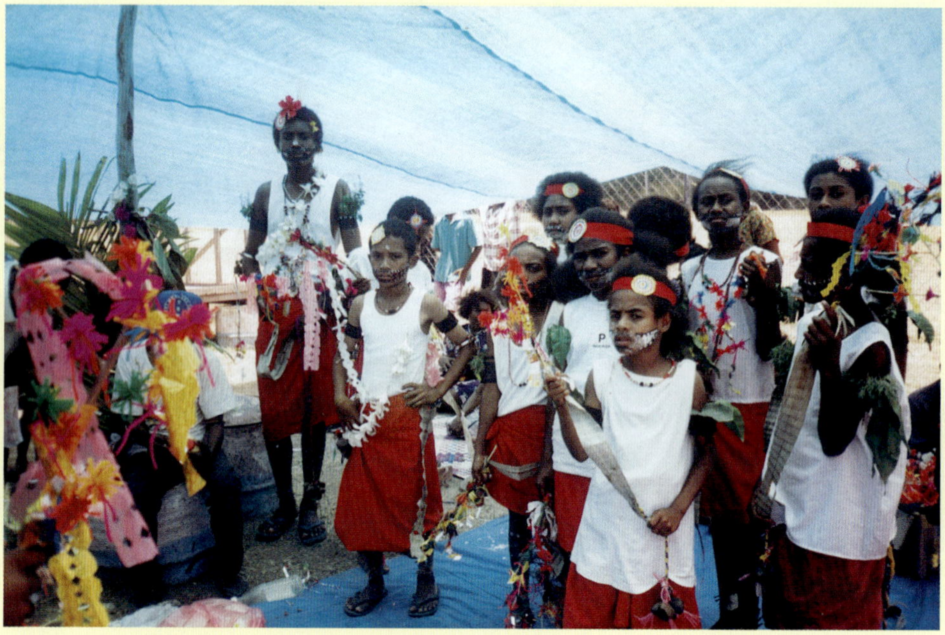

Behaviour that can lead to the breakdown of relationships

Sometimes the way that people behave means that the relationship starts to break down. Their behaviour may even lead to fighting. For example:

- when people get angry and cross and shout at each other
- when people stop cooperating with each other and oppose each other instead
- when people stop listening to each other
- when people deliberately make trouble
- when people try to shame others, or humiliate them or show disrespect

We should try to avoid this type of behaviour if we want our relationships with other people to be happy and successful.

For you to try

- Copy and complete the following table. One example has been completed for you. You can add more rows to the bottom of the table if you want to.

Ways to maintain a healthy relationship	Skills needed
Gather information that is needed	Observing and asking questions, listening carefully, checking
Communicate well with others	
Give and receive compliments (positive comments about each other)	
Solve problems	
Weigh up information, make a decision and then carry out the decision	
Other?	

- Think about two people, one you communicate well with and one you do not. Describe your relationship with each person and give reasons. Discuss ways to maintain or improve the relationship with each person.

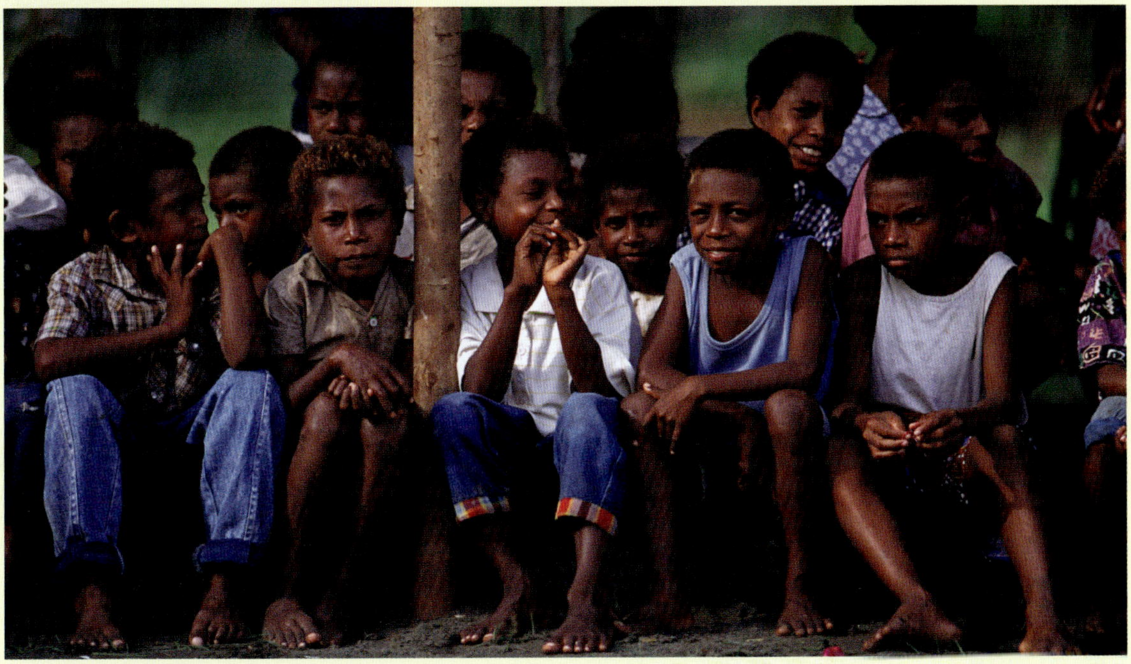

2

Movement and Physical Activity

Chapter Summary

In this chapter you will have an opportunity to:

- ✔ Learn to link movement skills that are used in games, sports and dance
- ✔ Learn different sequences of movements that demonstrate body control
- ✔ Find out more what it means to be fit and the activities that promote fitness
- ✔ Find out more about rules and safety procedures so as to prevent injury when we play
- ✔ Find out how to help people to take part in recreation leisure activities
- ✔ Find out more about the different roles and responsibilities in games and sport

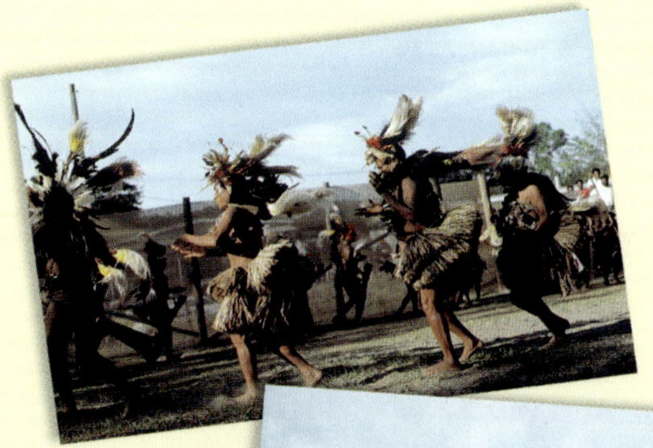

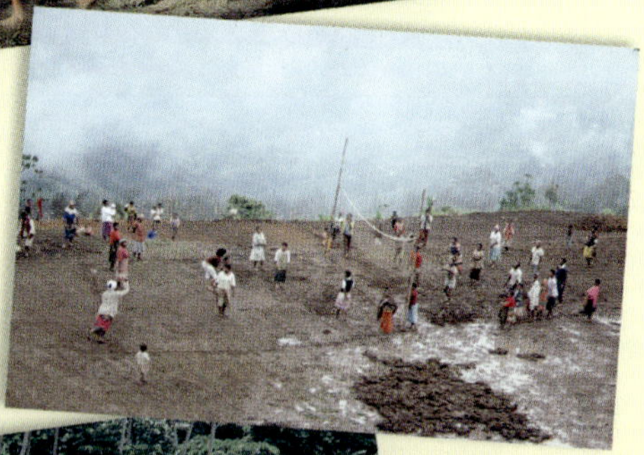

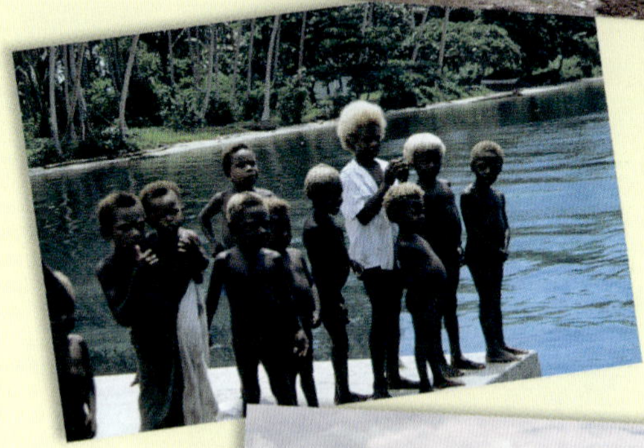

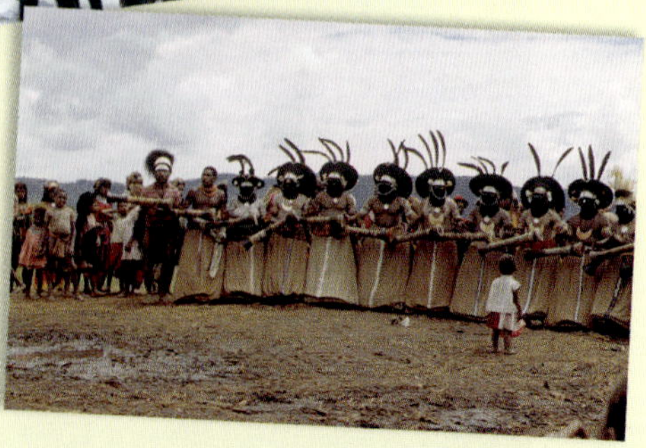

Syllabus references

Strand: Movement and physical activity
Sub-strands: Movement skills, fitness for health, safety, leisure and recreation, roles and responsibilities

Outcomes:

7.2.1 Link a series of locomotor and non-locomotor skills using equipment in games and sports

7.2.2 Perform movement skills that demonstrate body control

7.2.3 Participate in a variety of physical activities that contribute to the development of particular components of fitness

7.2.4 Develop procedures for dealing with unsafe emergency situations

7.2.5 Plan different strategies to promote participation in recreational and leisure activities

7.2.6 Describe how taking on different roles affects attitudes, relationships and behaviour

Movement skills

LINKING SIMPLE SKILLS

Key facts

- To take part in games, sports and dance we need to link a range of different skills together.
- When we learn sequences of movements we need to develop good body control.
- Taking part in a variety of physical activities helps to develop different parts of our fitness.
- Some sporting activities can be dangerous and we need to know how to deal with dangerous situations and with emergencies.
- In order to encourage people to take part in recreational and leisure activities, suitable plans are needed.
- In some games and in organised sport, there are different codes of behaviour for the various roles that people take.

In many sports and games we usually have to move about or move from one place to another place. When we move from place to place we say that we **travel.** These skills are called **locomotor skills** and we usually combine or link together several different skills. For example, we:

- combine running, jumping, hopping and skipping
- take off and land using one foot or two feet
- travel taking weight on different parts of the body such as the legs and feet, or maybe the arms and hands
- travel through water using different arm and leg actions

Some sports and games also need skills that do not involve travelling or moving from one place to another. These skills are called **non-locomotor skills**. For example, when you are dancing you might need to make rhythmic actions with your hands and feet, such as clapping your hands or clicking your fingers, but not move from the same spot. Other examples of non-locomotor skills are running on the spot, spinning, jumping, turning and twisting in your own personal space.

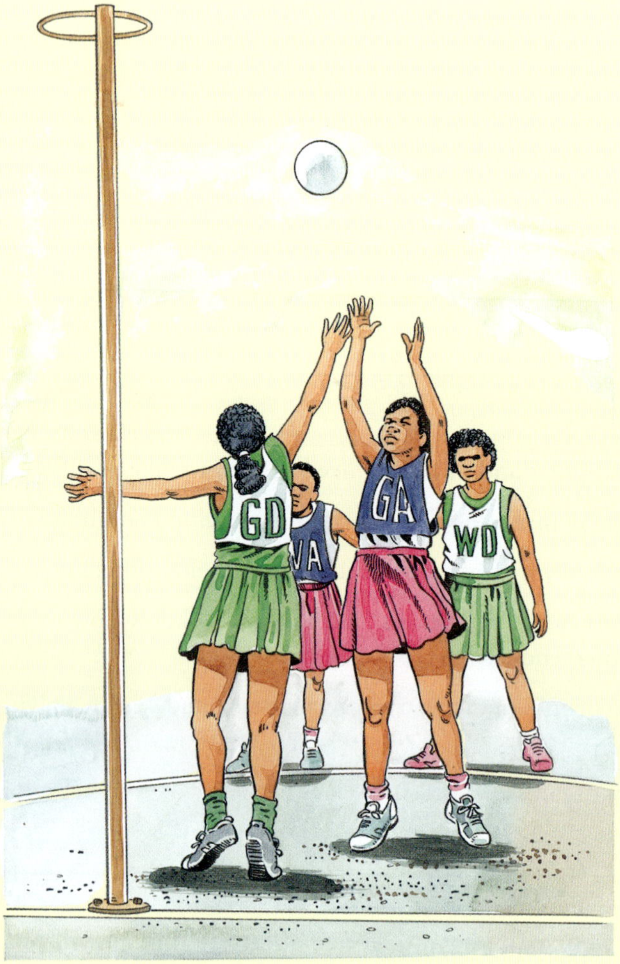

LINKING LOCOMOTOR AND NON-LOCOMOTOR SKILLS

In many sports and in games we need to combine the skills that allow us to move from place to place with other skills, such as hitting or catching a ball. For example, when playing volleyball we may need to move quickly around the court, but we also need to hit the ball so that it goes where we want it to go. When we play rugby we need to run but also to pass the ball backwards to the next player. Passing and receiving the ball without dropping it are important skills. During traditional dancing you need to be in the right position, but you might also be keeping time with a kundu drum or you might be making some other movements with your arms and hands.

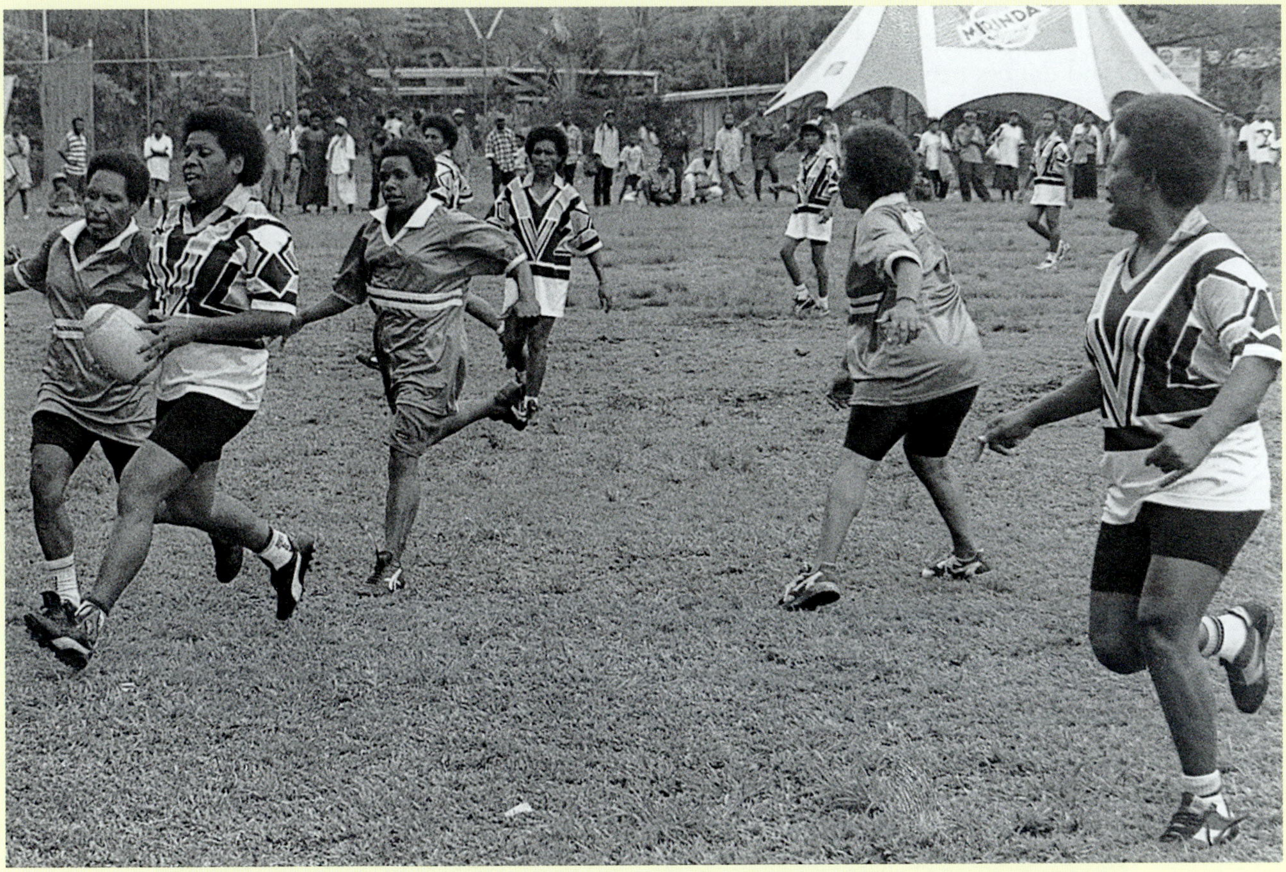

For you to try

- Practise skills such as running, hopping, skipping and jumping.
- Practise skills used in ball games such as throwing a ball, fielding a ball, catching a ball, passing a ball.
- Practise running and jumping and combine this with balancing—like walking along a piece of wood or balancing a ball.
- A Make up a game that includes skills that you learnt as a child and what you like to do now. Play the game with your friends. Change the skills and the rules if you like. For example, the egg and spoon race can be played using round nuts or seeds instead of eggs. You could hold the spoon in your mouth instead of in your hand.

MOVEMENT SKILLS THAT DEMONSTRATE BODY CONTROL

Many sports and dances need a number of different skills. We learn movement skills by observing, practising and building on these skills. Examples of skills that require body control are:

- to throw for speed, distance, accuracy and height
- to move to catch a ball or other object
- to balance on different parts of the body
- to perform set body actions in time to rhythm or music
- to turn or twist correctly during a body movement

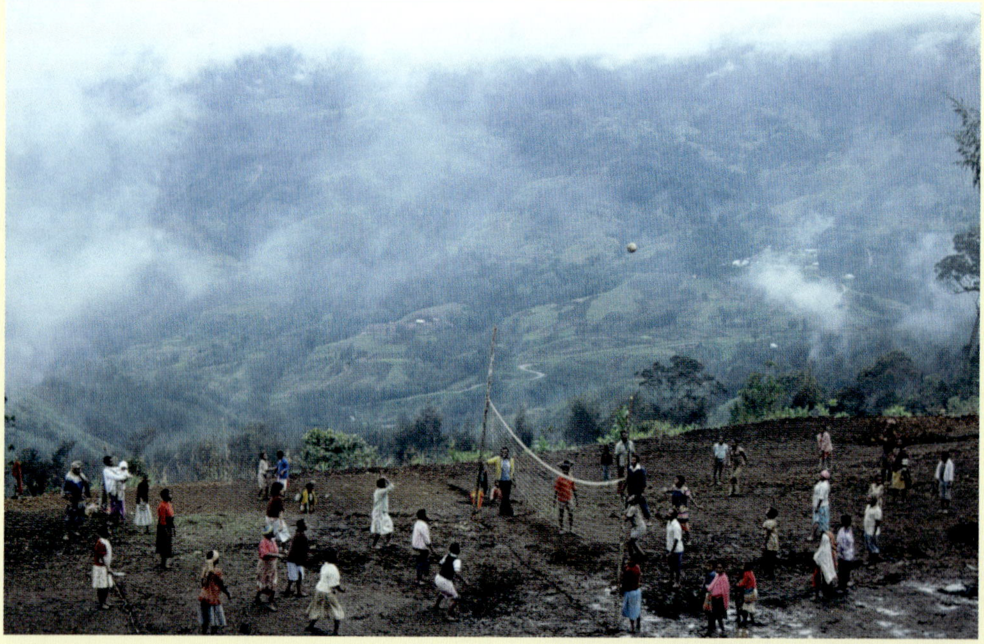

Fitness for health

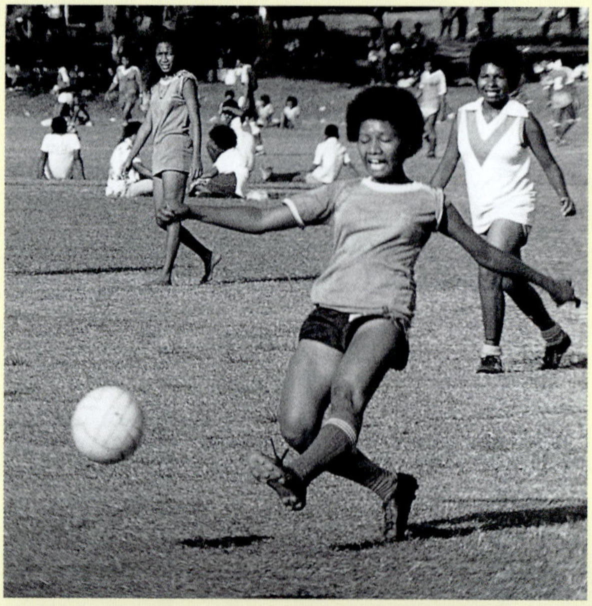

A healthy heart and lungs are needed to carry oxygen to the muscles which helps us to work and play without getting out of breath or getting tired too quickly. A healthy heart and lungs also help to prevent disease.

There are many activities that help us to be fit. Any activity that makes the heart pump faster and makes us breathe more quickly is healthy activity. Many of these are everyday activities like gardening, cutting grass, sweeping leaves and keeping the house and the community clean. Walking, running and swimming also help to make the heart and the lungs work well.

For you to try

- Choose skills from games that require body control and practise them. For example, throwing a ball, catching a ball, passing a ball, dribbling a ball with the feet or the hands, balancing.
- Play some simple team games that require body control and coordination. For example, tunnel ball, the egg and spoon race, three-legged race, balancing a piece of paper on the head while running as fast as possible. Think of some more of your own.

Regular **stretching** of the body is also important. Stretching the body helps the joints to be flexible. If we don't stretch the arms and the legs, then it becomes difficult to carry out some activities such as bending down to pick up something from the ground. Most Papua New Guineans can sit on the floor with their legs crossed for long periods of time because they regularly stretch their legs when they do this. People who do not usually sit with legs crossed may find it hard to stretch their legs in this way.

Lifting and carrying any weight also helps to build the strength of the muscles of the arms and legs and to increase our endurance so that we can continue doing the activity for as long as is needed.

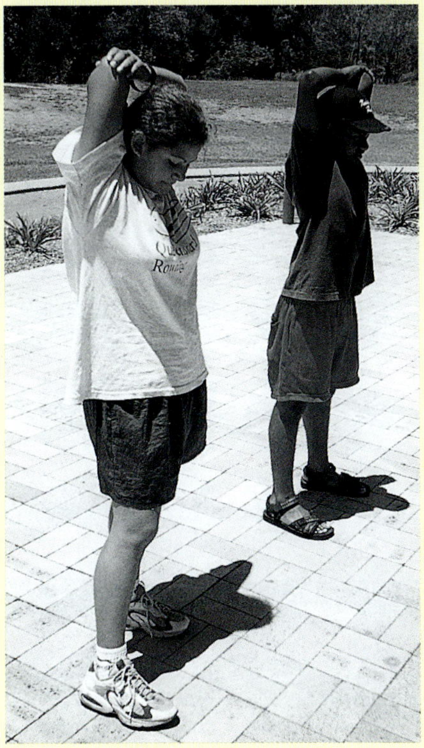

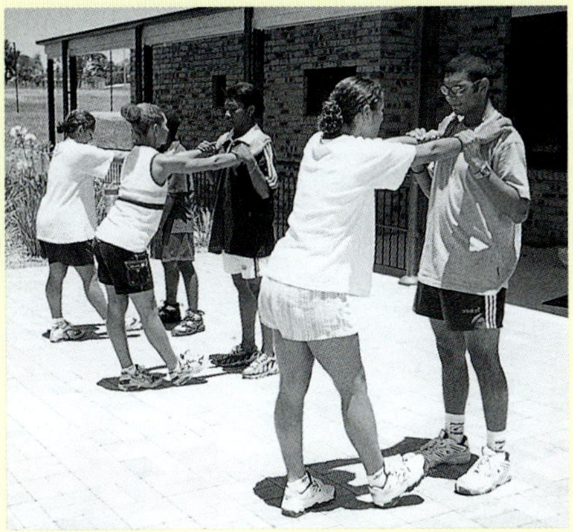

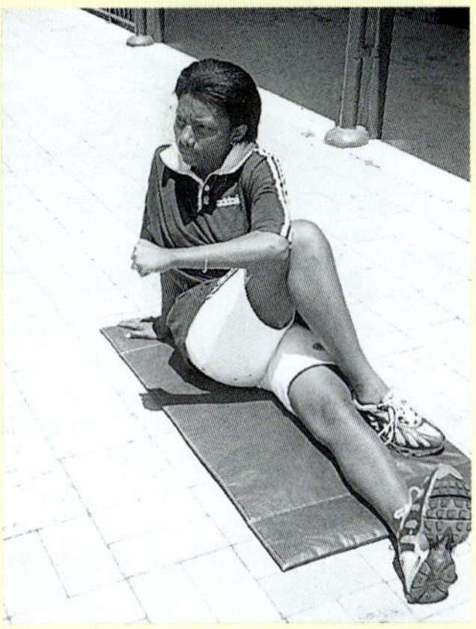

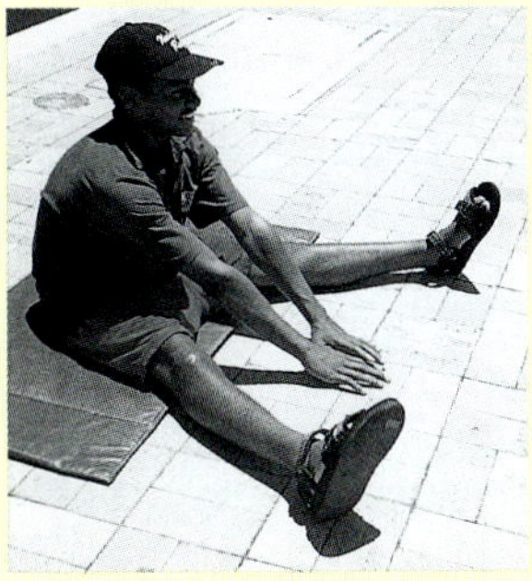

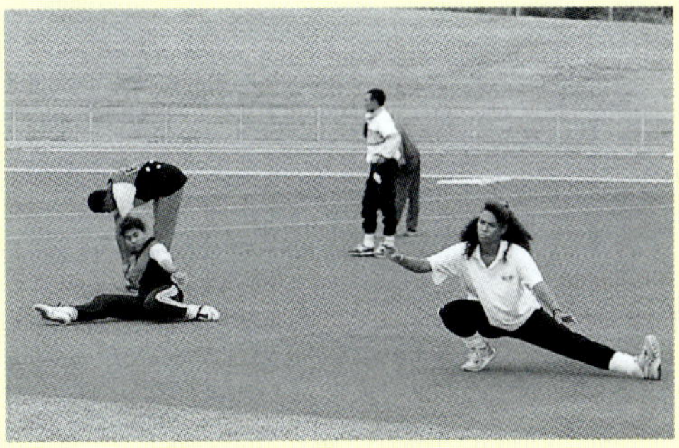

For you to try

- Copy and complete the following list of competitive and non-competitive physical activities in which you have taken part this year. Two examples have been given. Add as many rows as you need.

Non-competitive	Competitive
Sweeping leaves	Playing netball

A • Keep a diary or a log like the one below to show the activities that you take part in, and the amount of time you spend on each activity. Remember to include everyday activities as well as sports.

Date	Activity	Time spent on this activity
April 1	Playing April Fool's jokes on friends	30 minutes
	Cutting grass round school	
	Sweeping leaves	
	Swimming	
	Walking to school	

Compare your diary with your classmates' diaries.
Who has the biggest number of activities?
Who spends the most time on each activity?

ML Safety

SAFETY PROCEDURES

In order to keep yourself safe and to help others who may need help, you should learn how to deal with danger and emergency situations. For example:

- Learn to identify the risk or hazards to yourself or others.
- Have a plan to avoid risk and carry out your plan.
- Do not stay in a place where it feels unsafe or where there is fighting.
- Report fighting or abuse to someone that you trust.
- If it is safe to do so, try to help someone who is in difficulty. If you cannot help the person, go and get help from someone else.
- Learn basic first aid so that you can help someone who needs help.

TAKING RISKS

Whenever we play sport or take part in any physical activity, there is always a risk that we will get an injury or injure somebody else. We need to learn how to deal with some risks and avoid others. There are different types of risk and different ways that people take risks.

Some risk-taking behaviour helps the person to become a responsible person. For example, if we take a risk to help someone else who is having trouble or to prevent an accident, then this is positive risk-taking. Most people in the community would approve of this type of risk-taking. On the other hand, if we take a risk that could cause pain, injury or shame to someone else, then this is a negative risk. Most people in the community would not agree with this type of risk-taking.

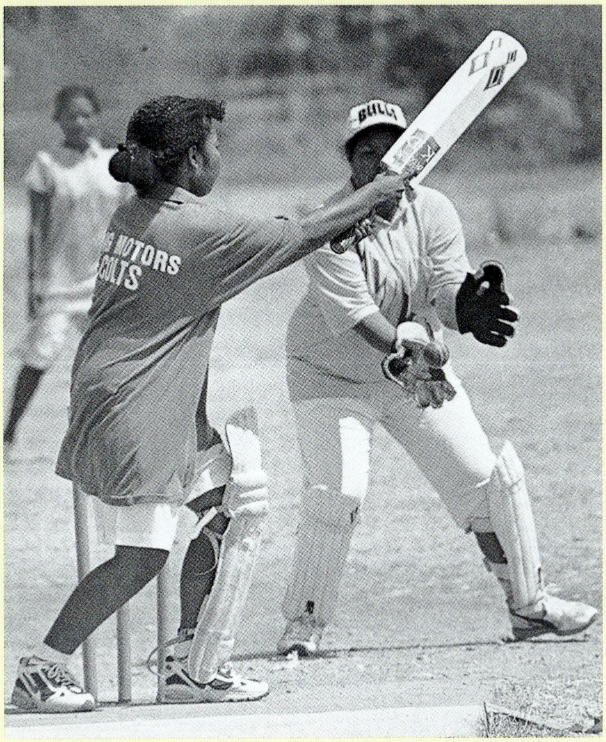

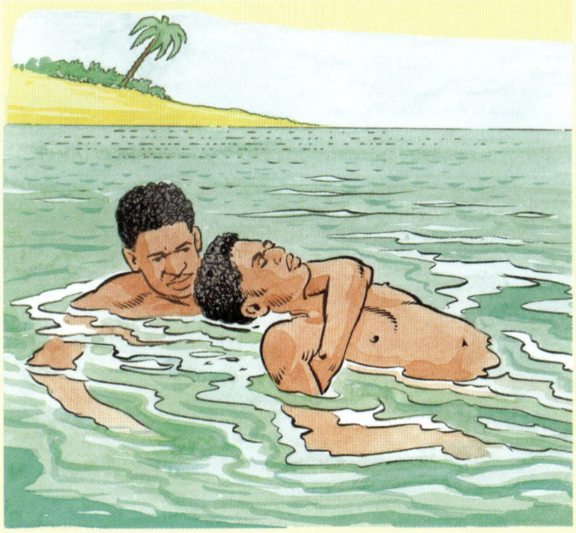

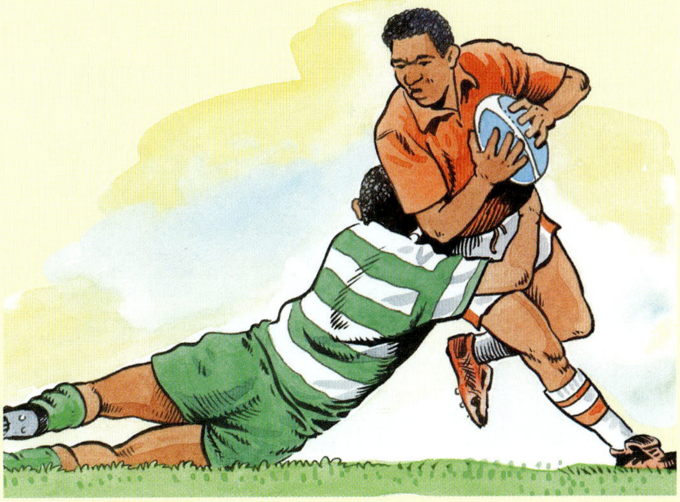

For you to try

- List three activities that you have taken part in recently that involved risks. Suggest how you could handle those risks to avoid accidents taking place.
- List the risks involved in a sport that you play. Write down how you can avoid the risk of injury.

Leisure and recreation

WAYS OF HELPING PEOPLE TO TAKE PART

Everyone needs to be encouraged to take part in activities that will help them to be healthy. Some groups may need extra help in order to allow them to take part.

Some things that we can do:

- Organise an activity for a selected group such as young students or people with disabilities.
- Think of ways to help girls and women to take a greater part in physical activity.
- Organise team competitions in games like netball, softball and volleyball.
- Organise sports as a way to build community relationships, not just for winning.
- Suggest ways that people can accept losing without getting angry.

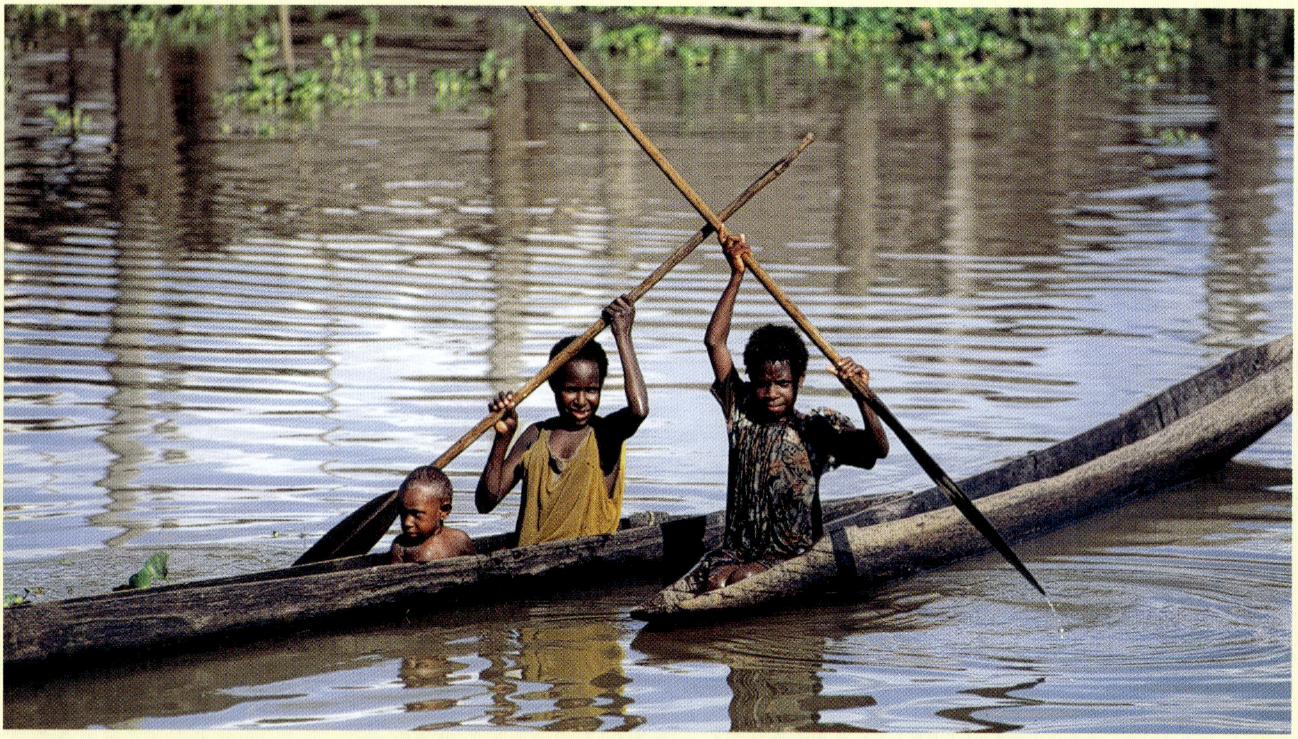

For you to try

- How can recreational activities be improved or promoted in your community? Design a questionnaire and interview different groups of people to answer these questions.
- Choose a group in your community that needs a leisure activity. Suggest ways to organise or improve a leisure activity for this group. Describe how it will benefit the community.

Sporting roles and responsibilities

CODES OF BEHAVIOUR FOR VARIOUS ROLES

In sport there are many different roles that people play in order for the sport to be played well and enjoyed by everyone. Some of these roles are player, captain, spectator, referee and coach. For each of these roles there is a code of behaviour that the person should follow.

- The players should play by the rules, play as a member of the team, take notice of the captain and the coach, and not fight.
- The spectators should support their team, accept the decisions of the referee, stay off the playing area and not fight.
- The referee should know and follow the rules of the game and be fair to both sides.
- The coach should help the players to develop their skills and fitness and should encourage fair play, discipline the players and try to prevent injuries.

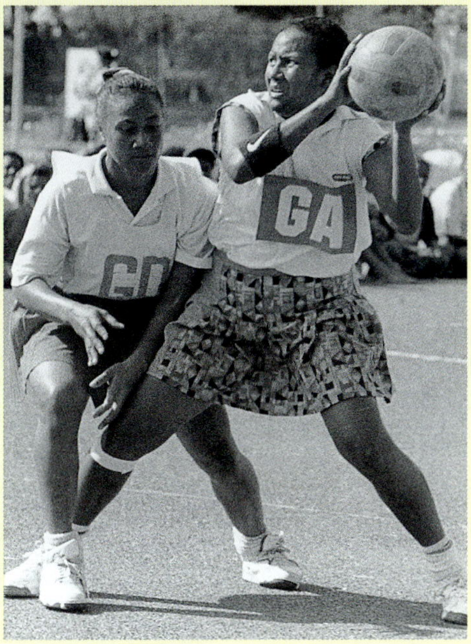

For you to try

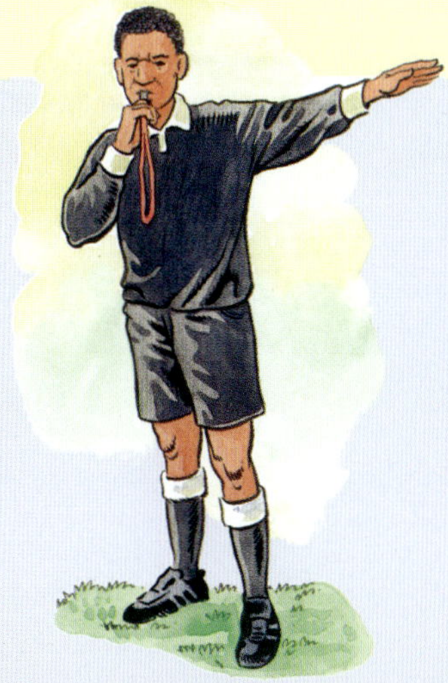

A Watch a game of sport or some other physical activity that is being performed by a group.

- Make a list of the roles and responsibilities that you observe.
- For each role, write a paragraph to describe how each role was carried out.
- Describe the strengths and the weaknesses of each role.
- Suggest ways to improve the weaknesses next time the game is played or the physical activity is performed.

3

Our Culture, Lifestyle and Values

Chapter Summary

In this chapter you will have an opportunity to:

- ✔ Find out about ways that we maintain cultural practices that are important in the community
- ✔ Find out about changes in the environment that are affecting the way that people live

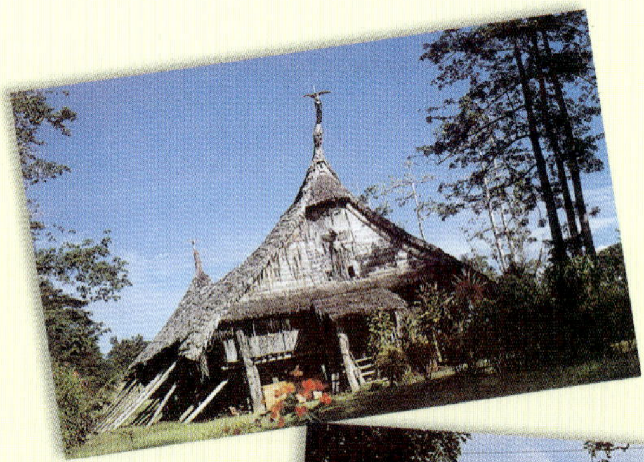

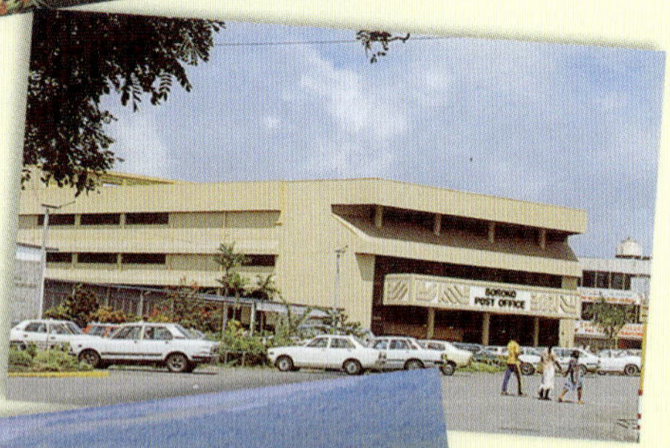

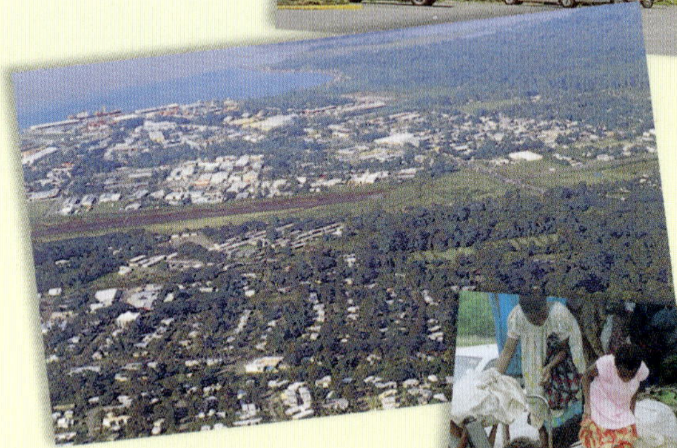

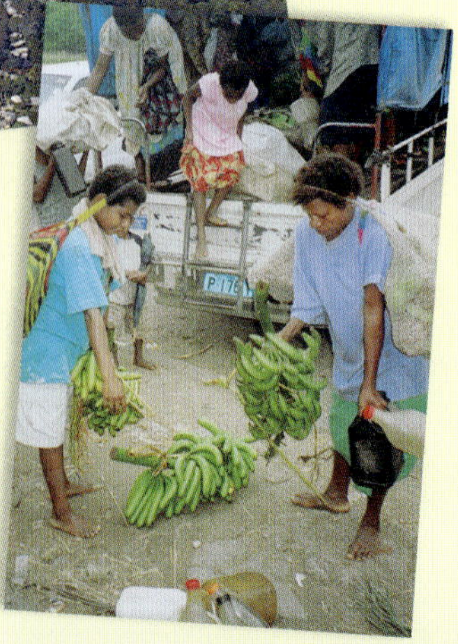

Syllabus references

Strand: Our culture, lifestyle and values
Sub-strands: Culture and values, lifestyle changes

Outcomes:

7.3.1 Discuss what can be done to maintain cultural practices valued by the community

7.3.2 Explore changes in the physical and economic environments and how they affect their lifestyle

Culture and values

MAINTAINING VALUED CULTURAL PRACTICES (ML)

Key facts

- Customs, rituals and traditions are still strong in Papua New Guinea but some may be lost or forgotten.
- There are many differences in the culture of people from different parts of the country.
- We should respect our own culture and that of people from other parts of the country and from other countries.
- Many changes are taking place to the way of life of people in Papua New Guinea and some of these are affecting the culture.

In Papua New Guinea, the culture of the people is still strong and people maintain their way of life in a number of different ways. For example, when people speak their own language they are practising an important part of their culture. There are Elementary Schools in many provinces in which the children are taught in their own language in the first three grades. This helps the students to learn more about their culture and to practise their language. Papua New Guinea is famous for having so many different languages—about 860 altogether.

Another part of culture is the way that people dress. When we see people in traditional dress, or we see a photograph, we can usually tell if they are from the Highlands or from the New Guinea Islands or from the Papuan coast. You can probably even guess which province they are from.

Food is another important part of the culture, especially the **staple food** that people eat every day. Sweet potato, yams, taro, sago and bananas are all examples of staple foods in different parts of Papua New Guinea. Rice has also become an important food for many people and is a staple food for millions of people in Asian countries. When people move away from their own area, one of the things that they miss most is the food from their place.

One of the ways that people keep their culture alive is by performing dances on important occasions in the village, at school celebrations and provincial shows.

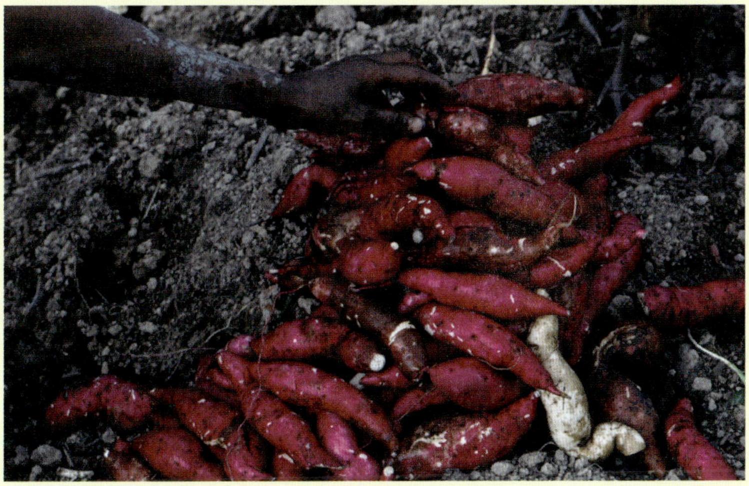

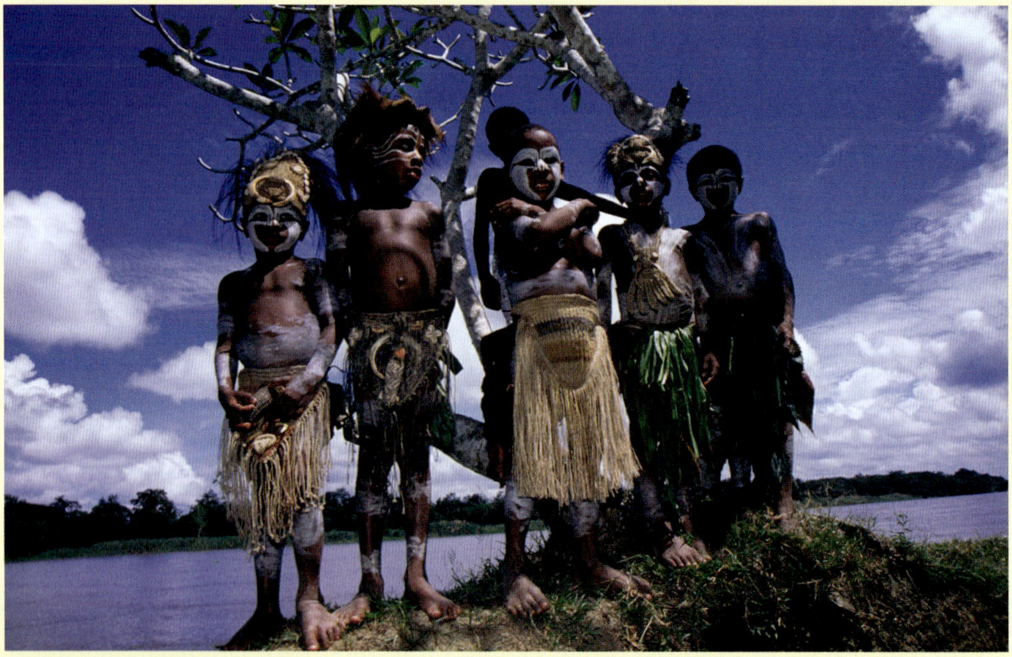

CELEBRATIONS AND THEIR IMPORTANCE

Celebrations help to develop feelings of being part of the community. For example, everyone in Papua New Guinea celebrates New Year's Day, the Queen's Birthday in June and the anniversary of independence on September 16. Then there are different days celebrated by each province.

People from different religions also celebrate different beliefs. For example, Christmas and Easter are two important festivals for Christians to celebrate. Jewish people celebrate Passover, which begins in late March or early April and lasts for eight days. Muslim people do not eat or drink between sunrise and sunset for a month during Ramadan. This practice is called fasting. Children do not have to fast.

For you to try

- Describe the cultural customs and beliefs for your area or an area you know well that are associated with food preparation, gardening, fishing, dancing, birth and pregnant mothers.
- Identify a cultural belief or practice that is slowly disappearing and give reasons for this (for example, traditional clothing).
- Conduct a survey to find out the cultural customs and beliefs for an area that is not yours, or that you do not know well.
- Some customs, beliefs or other cultural practices are valued more than others. Find out about the reasons why this is so.
- Explain how cultural practices can be maintained or improved.

Lifestyle and changes

CHANGES IN THE ENVIRONMENT ML SS

There have been many changes to the surroundings or environment in Papua New Guinea. For example, one of the important changes is the way in which people build their houses. Although there are still many houses made from bush materials, people also like to use materials such as corrugated iron. People like corrugated iron because it is easy to use, lasts for a long time and can be used to collect rainwater for drinking. However, corrugated iron is more expensive, and a house with an iron roof is hotter than one made from bush materials. In other words, changes can be *positive* or *negative*.

There have been many other changes in different provinces. For example:

- roads that allow people to move about more easily, to buy and sell goods and to reach schools and hospitals
- new crops and farming methods that increase the variety of food and allow people to earn money (for example, rubber, coffee, oil palm)
- electricity that can be used for lights, cooking and refrigerators
- a clean water supply that makes life easier and helps to keep people healthy
- new schools, hospitals and health centres
- land cleared for logging or mining (which can also cause damage to land, rivers and wildlife, and loss of farming land)

Changes to the environment can be of three types—**physical, economic** and **social**. Physical change means a change in the appearance of the surroundings. Economic change means a change in the way that people buy and sell goods and make businesses. Social change means a change in the way that people live together in the community.

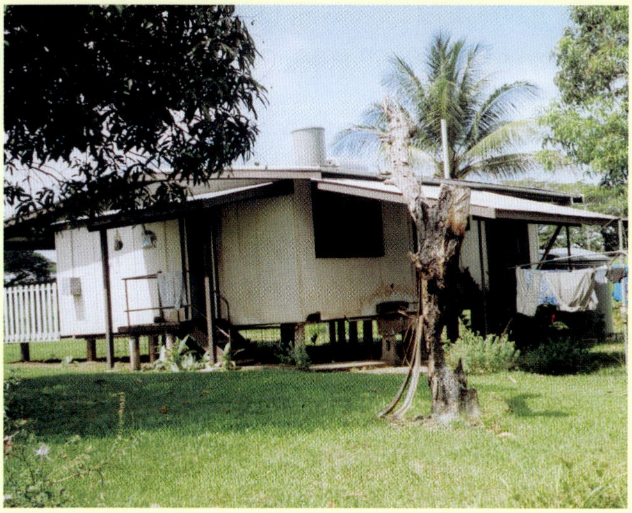

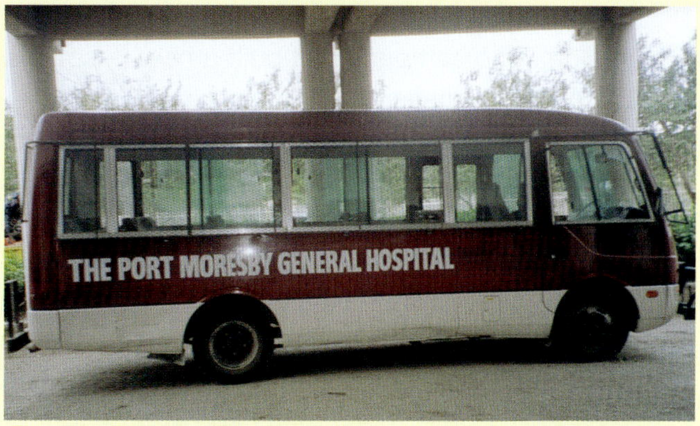

Moale comes to town

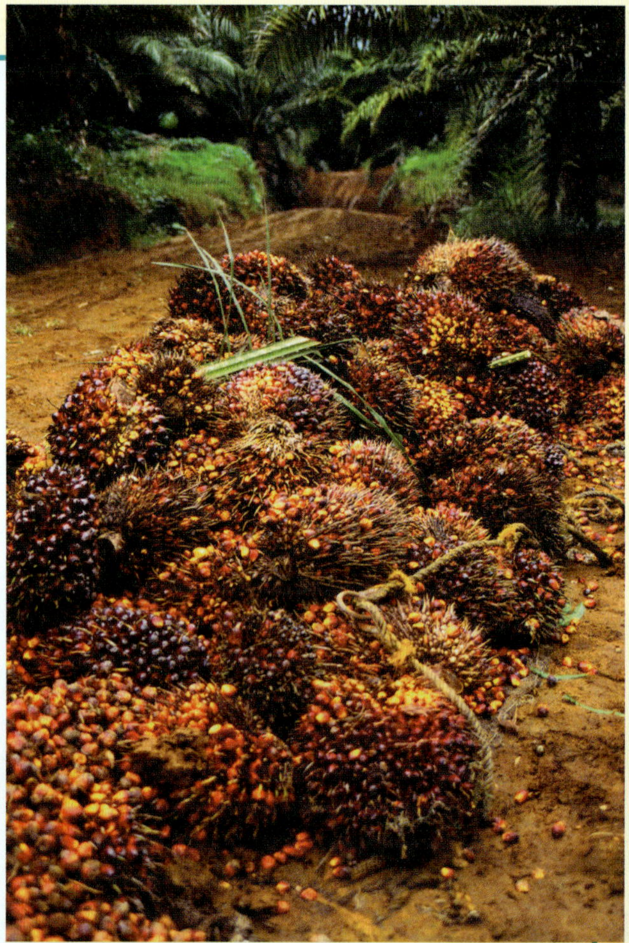

Oil palm nuts on the side of the road

Moale was beginning to notice the changes taking place in her province. Near her village the old coconut plantation had been sold to a big company and it had knocked down all the old coconuts and planted oil palm. The lovely river where people used to swim, catch prawns and have picnics was now churned up by big machines that drove through making the water muddy. There had already been some road accidents, and soon there would be many trucks driving up and down the road carrying the palm oil to the wharf.

Further over the hill there was a new timber project. One of the men who worked for the company said that they were cutting down some of the biggest trees he had ever seen in his life. Moale felt sad about this, but the new road did help people to get to town more easily. There was also a story going round that there were not as many big trees as the company had expected and the project might not last for many years. If this happened, the people would not be paid as much money as they had been promised.

Moale's uncle was working for a new mine that had started in a different part of the province. The company knew that the mine had a life of only a few years, but it did provide some jobs (although many of the special jobs went to people from outside). The company had built a new hospital but there was not enough equipment or enough doctors and nurses.

In the town there were not just the usual Chinese stores but also a department store where you could buy almost everything that you needed—as long as you had the money in your pocket. Some children had been caught stealing because they did not have the money to buy the nice things that they could see in the new store.

There was also a new market building, and more village people were bringing fruit and vegetables to sell to the people who had come to work in the province. The village people enjoyed the extra money they could earn, but there was also more trouble in the town, especially on pay weekends. Some young men had been caught drinking by the police and some local women said that they no longer felt safe at night.

Moale thought about all these changes and wondered what life would be like in her province in the future. 'How can we take the good changes without having too many problems?' she wondered.

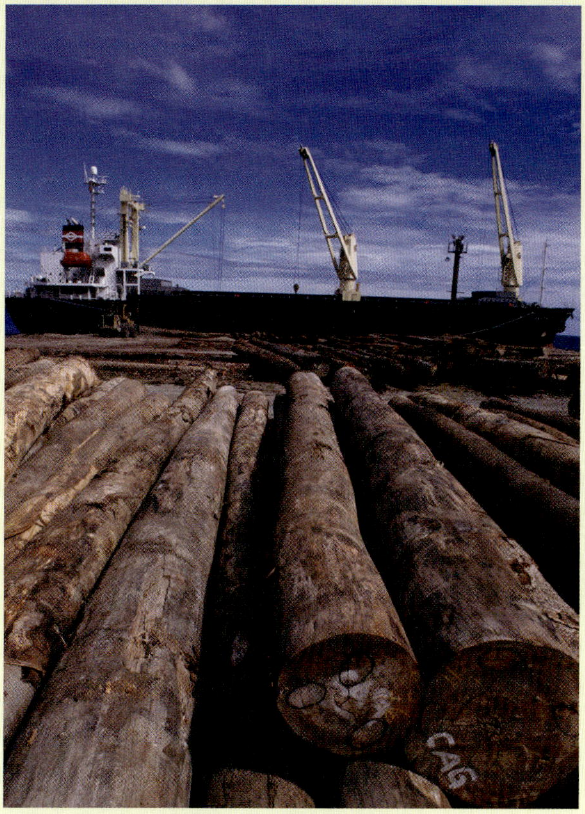

Logging forest trees for export

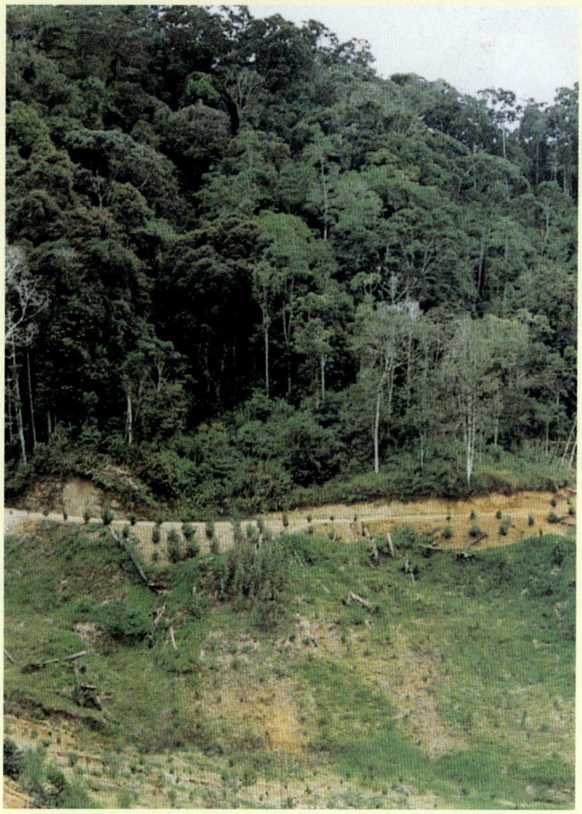
Reforestation at Mount Victoria

For you to try

- Make groups of four or five students. Discuss the changes that have taken place in the environment in your community. Make a list of these changes and say whether you think each change is positive or negative.
- Choose a change that has taken place in your community, or one that is taking place now. Explain how the change can have a positive and a negative effect on the lifestyle of people in the community.
- Read the story 'Moale comes to town'. List all the changes that are taking place under three headings:

Physical	Economic	Social

How can Moale and the people in her province take the good changes without having the problems that come with these changes?

4

Health of Individuals and Population

Chapter Summary

In this chapter you will have an opportunity to:

- ✔ Find out about different parts of the body and the way they work
- ✔ Find out about the changes that happen as we grow up
- ✔ Find out about different behaviour that can increase or reduce the respect that we have for each other
- ✔ Find out about different food and ways of eating among different people
- ✔ Plan healthy meals using local food
- ✔ Make a personal health plan
- ✔ Learn how to deal with situations that are unsafe and unhealthy
- ✔ Learn ways that keep you safe and healthy
- ✔ Find out more about how we can help the community to be healthy
- ✔ Find out how the environment is being changed because of development and how this can affect our health
- ✔ Find out more about the effect of using drugs in the community
- ✔ Learn ways to make your own decisions and to follow them through

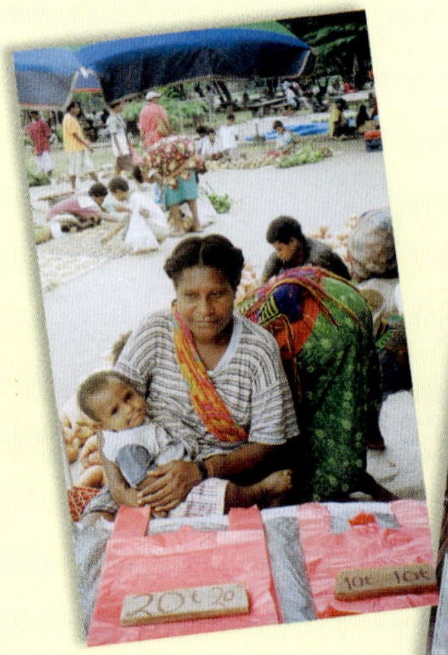

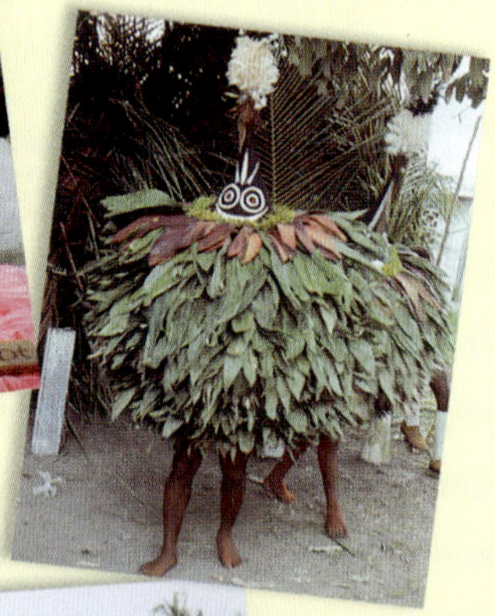

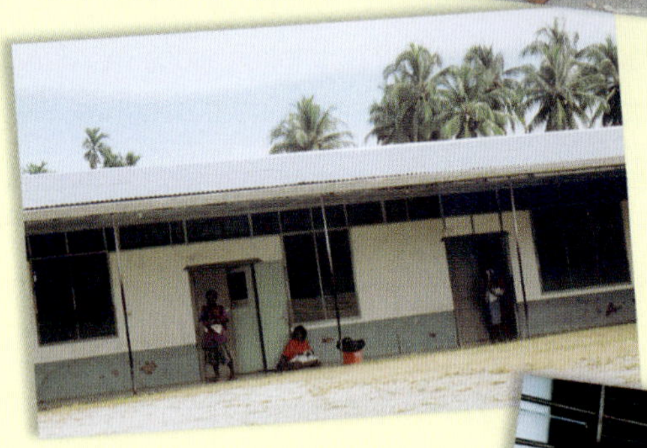

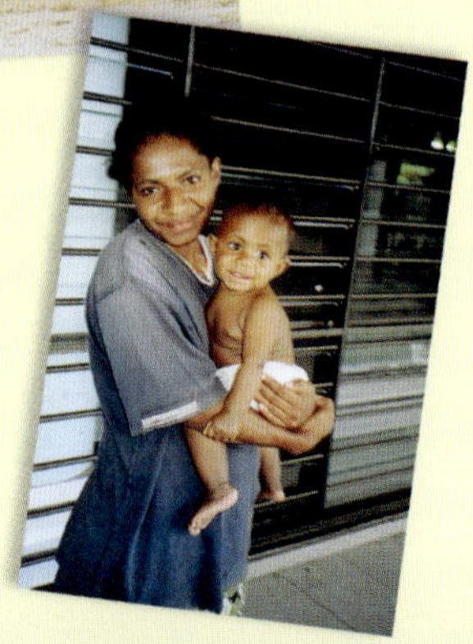

Syllabus references

Strand: Health of individuals and population
Sub-strands: Growth and development, nutrition, personal health and safety, community health, use of drugs

Outcomes:

7.4.1 Explore the functions of different systems and parts of the body

7.4.2 Describe the physical, social and emotional changes in both boys and girls during puberty

7.4.3 Identify situations and behaviour relating to the human body and how these behaviours promote or lessen respect for individuals and groups

7.4.4 Explain why groups and individuals in the same community may have different eating and meal patterns

7.4.5 Plan meals to meet nutritional needs using locally available food

7.4.6 Develop a personal health plan based on a personal health goal

7.4.7 Propose ways of responding to situations that threaten personal health and safety

7.4.8 Describe behaviours that affect personal community safety

7.4.9 Describe basic concepts and methods of health promotion and illness prevention in the community

7.4.10 Investigate how the environment is being changed by human behaviour and development and the effect of these changes on health

7.4.11 Describe decisions people make about drug use and the result of those decisions on the community and the individuals

7.4.12 Propose ways of responding to pressures to use harmful substances

Key facts

- The main purpose of the reproductive system is to allow men and women to have children.
- When we grow up from girls into women and from boys into men, many changes take place in our appearance and in the way that we feel and behave.
- The way that we behave can increase or reduce the respect that we have for each other.
- Eating is a behaviour that varies among people from different places. People eat different kinds of food and eat in different ways.
- Everyone can plan healthy and nutritious meals using food that is available locally.
- We can make plans and choices about our own health using our knowledge about what makes us sick.
- We can keep ourselves healthy by avoiding drugs and other risky situations that threaten our personal health and safety.
- Our behaviour should not have a negative effect on the health of other people in the community.
- We can help others in the community to learn about health and safety and to prevent illness.
- Because of the ways that we live, we are having an effect on the environment which in turn is having an effect on our health.
- Drugs can affect the health of people who use them and also have a negative effect on other people in the community.
- Each person has a choice about whether he or she will use drugs and alcohol.

Growth and development

PUBERTY AND ADOLESCENCE

As you grow up, your body changes and you become sexually mature. This means that you are able to reproduce or have children. The age when this stage is reached varies, but it is usually between the ages of ten and seventeen. Girls usually start to become sexually mature about two years earlier than boys. The stage in life when a child develops into an adult is called **puberty**.

The time between puberty and being a mature adult is known as adolescence. During adolescence you learn to think and behave as an adult. Adolescence can last for ten years or more and can be a difficult time for some young people, their parents and teachers. During this time you may find that your feelings are mixed up and your moods change quickly.

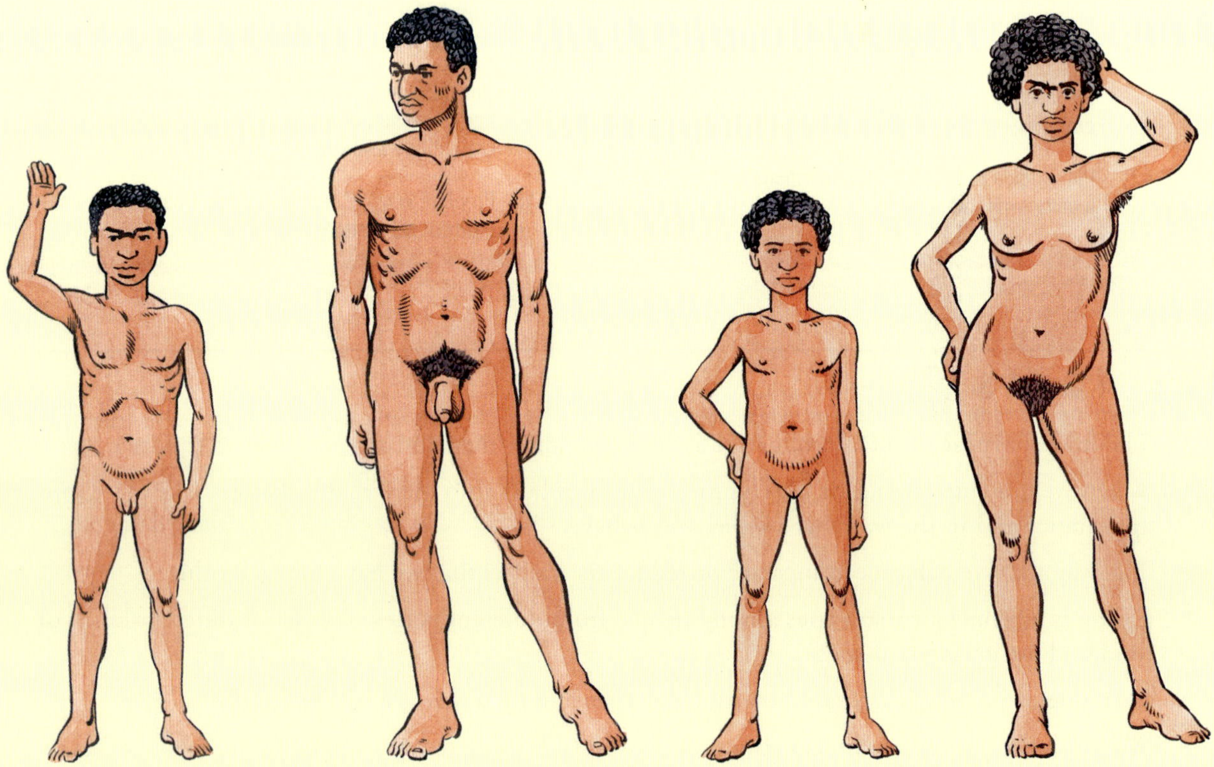

During puberty a girl's body becomes taller and heavier. The hips become wider, the breasts develop and the internal sex organs start to grow. The hips and bottom also become fatter. Hair begins to grow in the armpits and in the **pubic area**. The most important change is that ovaries start to produce eggs. The egg can develop into a baby when fertilised. If the egg is not fertilised it passes out of the vagina with some blood. This flow of blood is called a **period** or **menstruation** and happens about every four weeks. Periods are a normal thing to happen and the girl should not feel ashamed.

Some girls have pains when they have their periods and find that they feel differently before or during a period. For example, a girl might feel worried, get cross or be more easily upset at these times. These different moods can occur because of the chemical changes taking place inside her body. They are a normal thing to happen and the girl should not be worried about them. These feelings should be understood by the girl and by others who live with her.

During puberty a boy's body becomes taller and heavier. The shoulders and chest grow wider, the voice becomes deeper and the penis becomes bigger. Hair begins to grow in the armpits, in the pubic area and on the face. The most important change is that that the **testicles** or balls begin to produce **sperm**. The purpose of sperm is to fertilise the egg, which will then grow into a baby. When a boy starts to produce sperm it means that it is possible for him to become a father. Sperm are carried out of the penis in special liquid called **semen**.

Sometimes when a boy is asleep, semen passes out of his penis. When this happens it is called a **wet dream**. Wet dreams happen from time to time with no regular time interval between them. A wet dream is a normal thing to happen and the boy should not feel ashamed about it.

THE MALE REPRODUCTIVE SYSTEM (S)

At puberty the testicles begin to produce sperm. A man produces millions of tiny sperm throughout his life. The testicles or balls hang outside the body in a bag of skin called the **scrotum**. The scrotum is slightly cooler than the rest of the body which helps to produce healthy sperm. Two tubes called **sperm ducts** lead to the urethra. The urethra is the tube inside the penis that carries sperm and urine outside the body. The sperm are carried in milky-white liquid called semen. During sexual intercourse, the penis is placed inside the vagina and semen passes out through the urethra in the penis.

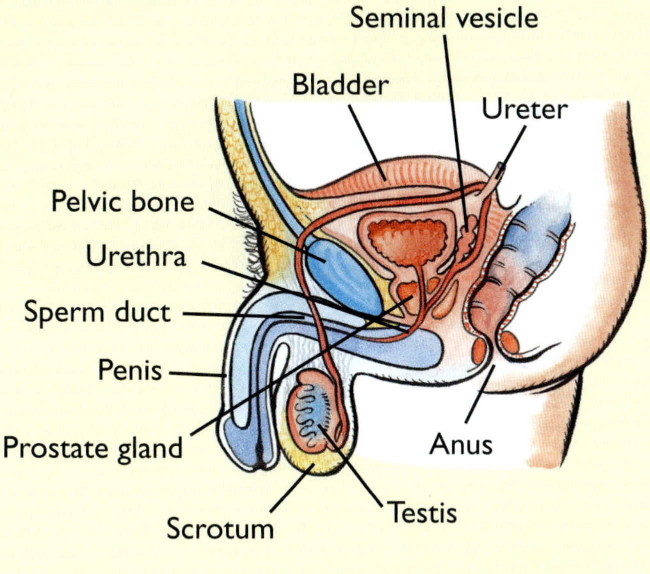

Side view

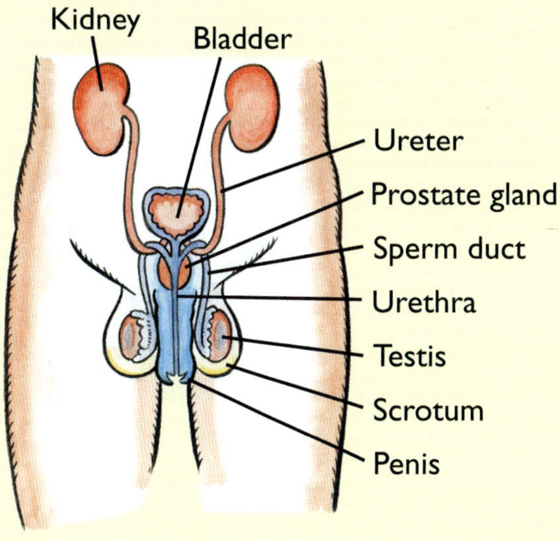

Front view

THE FEMALE REPRODUCTIVE SYSTEM (S)

At puberty the ovaries begin to release eggs. This will happen until the periods stop, which is usually when the woman is between the ages of forty and fifty. Usually one egg is produced each month from one of the ovaries. The egg travels down the oviduct or **Fallopian tube** towards the uterus. The uterus is the place where the baby develops. Before the egg is released, the uterus grows a special lining to receive it in case it is fertilised. If the egg is fertilised by a sperm in the oviduct, it moves down into the uterus and begins to grow into a baby. **Fertilisation** is also called **conception**.

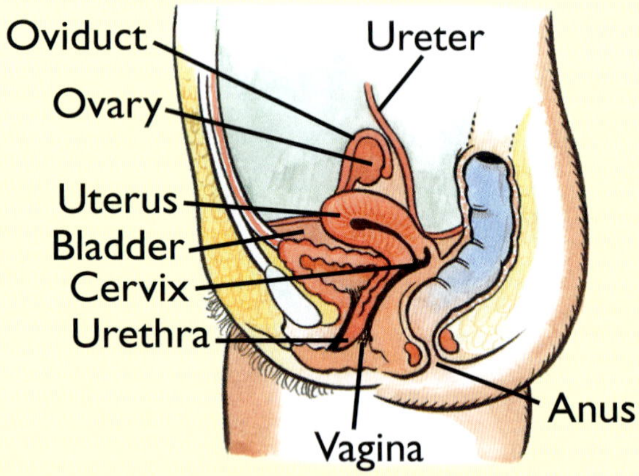

Side view

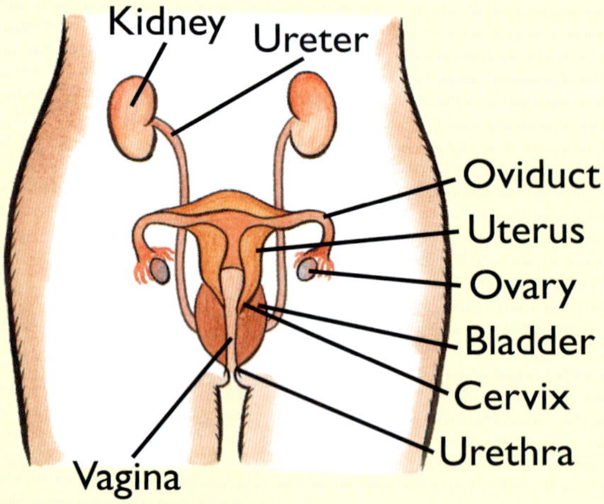

Front view

If the egg is not fertilised it will die after one or two days and later pass out of the body. The lining of the uterus continues to grow for several days. It then begins to break up and eventually leaves the body through the vagina during a period, which lasts about four or five days.

Traditionally, women in Papua New Guinea use leaves or dry grass to absorb the flow of blood. Modern methods use material napkins, cotton pads and tampons.

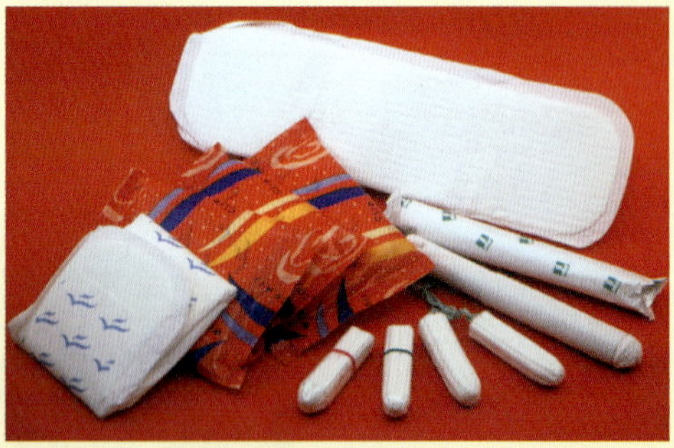

CHANGES DURING PUBERTY

As well as the physical changes that take place during puberty there are also social and emotional changes. Most young people find that the following happen:

Social changes

- You become more closely involved with friends or peers.
- You become more independent in the way that you think and behave.
- You experiment with new types of relationships, like having a boyfriend or girlfriend.
- You develop a sense of your own sexuality—the way that you think and feel and behave as a young man or young woman.
- You develop values, beliefs and behaviour which may be influenced by traditional ideas about what it means to be a man or a woman.

Lala's time

It happened when Lala was in Grade 7. She was sitting in class when her period came and left a stain on her skirt. She didn't know that it was going to happen, and so she wasn't prepared.

Sam, one of the boys who was sitting nearby, noticed what had happened and started to tell some of the other boys. They began looking at her and laughing, even though their teacher had explained that they should not do that. Soon the whole class seemed to know about it, although it was none of their business. Lala felt very embarrassed and just wanted to run away.

The other girls in the class also felt shy because they understood how she felt. Later on, when they were talking about it, all the girls agreed that it was wrong that the boys should make them feel shy about something that is a normal part of growing up and becoming an adult. 'It just shows that the boys haven't grown up yet,' one of the girls said.

For you to try

- Explain what is meant by puberty and adolescence.
- Describe the changes that take place in boys and girls at puberty.
- What are the similarities and differences between having a wet dream and having a period?
- Read the case study 'Lala's time' and answer the questions that follow:
  - — What should Lala do in this situation?
  - — What should Sam do?
  - — What should Lala's friends do?

Emotional changes

When you are an adolescent you will probably find that you experience very strong emotions. For example, some young people may find that the following happen:

- They love some things and some people, but hate others.
- They have very strong likes and dislikes.
- They feel very aggressive and want to argue with people.
- They have strong ideals and views about the way that things should be or the way that other people behave.
- They become very critical of other people.
- They get into arguments very easily.

One of the reasons for these changes is because of the hormones or chemicals in the body which control our physical development. Adolescence can be difficult for some people, but as we move through this time our bodies settle down and we learn to deal with many different situations without getting upset or angry.

For you to try

- List the physical, social and emotional changes in males and females during adolescence.
- With a group of friends, discuss how to manage the changes that take place in puberty.

ML RESPECT FOR INDIVIDUALS AND GROUPS

Respect is the way that we treat other people and the way that they treat us. Most people want to be respected both as individuals and as a group. Some behaviour that helps to encourage respect is as follows:

- greeting someone by smiling and shaking hands
- listening to different points of view
- accepting that there can be more than one correct answer or more than one way of doing something—not just your way
- putting other people first by helping them
- comforting or caring for people who are sick or old
- being humble and not putting yourself above other people

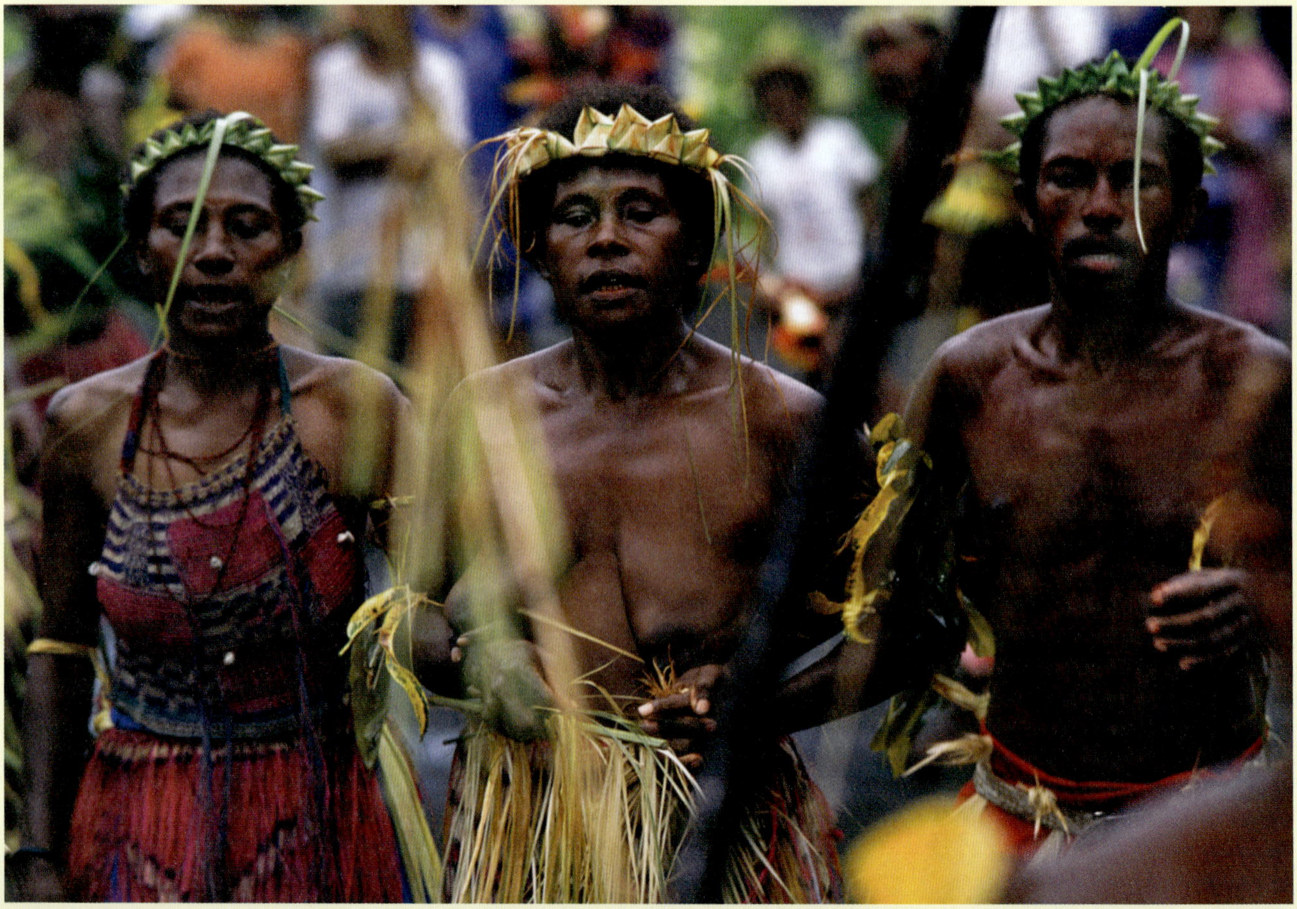

Some behaviour that reduces respect is as follows:

- shouting or using bad language
- calling people names
- refusing to talk about important issues
- interrupting other people and not letting them give their point of view
- being selfish and trying to get the best for yourself
- being aggressive and wanting to fight
- agreeing to do something and then not doing it

Influences on our behaviour

The way that people treat each other varies from one community to another and there are many influences on our behaviour. Our behaviour will be influenced by

- our values
- our parents
- our religious beliefs
- what we expect to gain from the behaviour
- other groups in the community
- how rich and powerful we are

For you to try

A • Work with a partner to copy and complete the following table:

My behaviour towards other people

Behaviour that encourages respect	Behaviour that reduces respect

- Write down some ways that you could improve behaviour that reduces respect.
- Think of a negative behaviour that you would like to change. Explain one reason that prevents you from changing.

Nutrition

CHOICES OF FOOD

The type of food that people eat and the way that it ;is cooked is one of the most important differences between people from different countries and from different provinces or regions of the same country. For most people, being able to get the kind of food that they like and having it cooked in ways that they like is a part of their identity.

Some reasons for the choice of food are:

- the availability of food
- the cost of food
- the time taken to prepare the food
- cultural and religious beliefs, practices and taboos
- the nutritional needs of different age groups, like young children, pregnant women or old people
- pressure from other people such as peers.

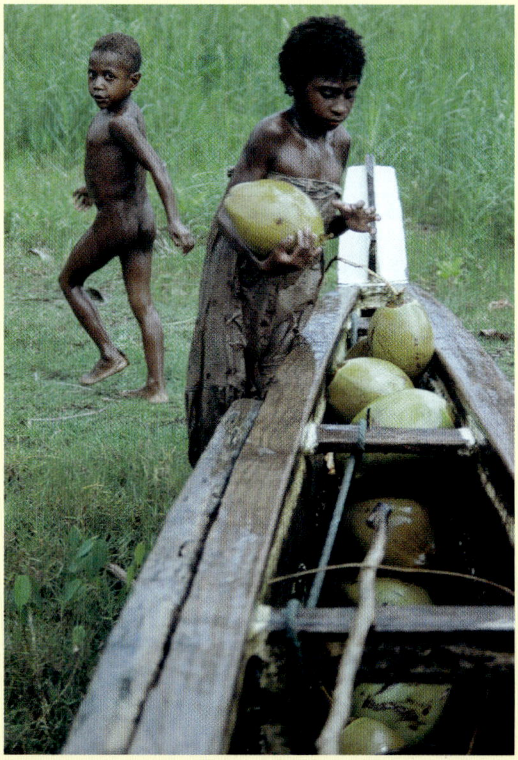

HEALTH PROBLEMS RELATED TO FOOD

The type and the amount of food that we eat also affects our health. All children and adults need to eat enough of the right kind of food every day. This is called eating a **balanced diet**.

When we do not eat enough of the right kind of food we feel hungry and eventually we will get sick. When children do not eat enough of the right kind of food they have **malnutrition.** Malnutrition is very common in Papua New Guinea and children who are malnourished are always underweight. Malnourished children also get infections easily and die more easily than other children.

If we eat too much of some types of food then we may become **overweight** or get other types of sickness. People who are very overweight suffer from obesity and are called **obese**. Being overweight or obese is unhealthy and can lead other health problems. Overweight and obesity are health problems that are beginning to happen to people living in towns in Papua New Guinea.

Some types of food can cause particular health problems. For example,

- Foods and drinks that contain a lot of sugar can cause tooth decay.
- Foods that contain a lot of animal fat or grease can make it hard for blood to move around the body.
- Foods that contain a lot of salt can cause high blood pressure.

The way that food is cooked or prepared is also important. For example, food that is fried contains more fat, and some foods contain extra sugar and salt. Eating food that contains a lot of fat and sugar or salt is not healthy. We should only eat these foods occasionally.

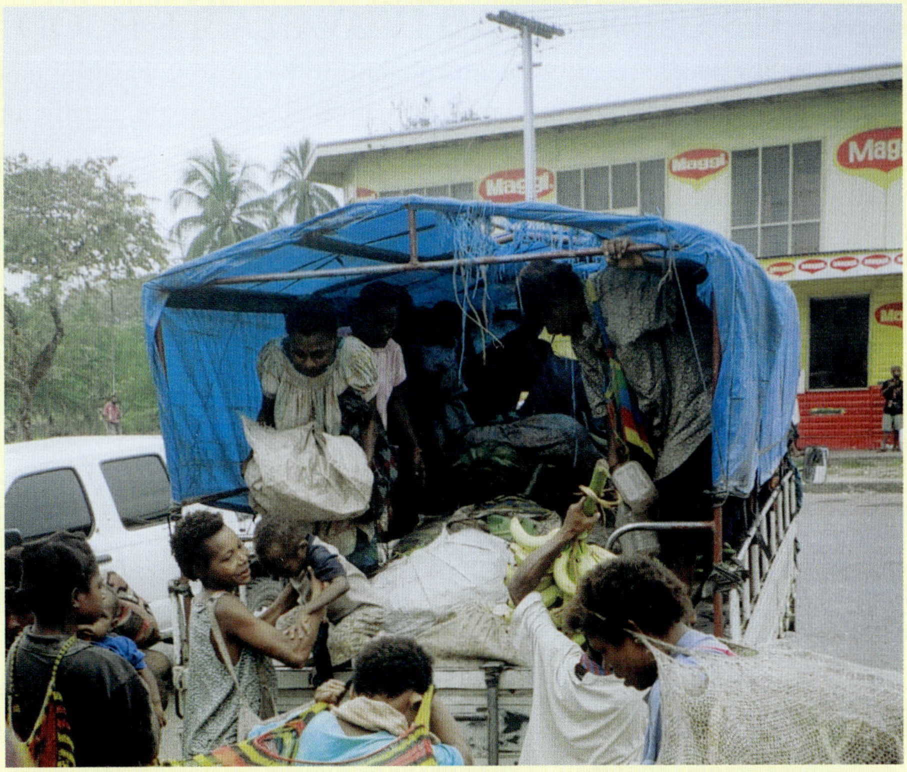

Traditional foods in Papua New Guinea do not contain extra sugar, fat or salt and so are healthy. Many Western foods—such as soft drinks, deep fried food and potato chips—contain extra sugar, fat or salt. People can get sick from eating these Western foods and this is beginning to happen to some people living in Papua New Guinea, especially in urban areas. However, when people go back to their traditional diet, this usually helps them to become healthy again.

Some foods like sweet potato and aibika contain a lot of **fibre**. Fibre is important because it allows the digestive system to work properly and helps us to go to the toilet. If you do not have enough fibre in your diet, and eat too much white bread, white rice and white sugar, you may become **constipated** and it will be hard to pass your faeces.

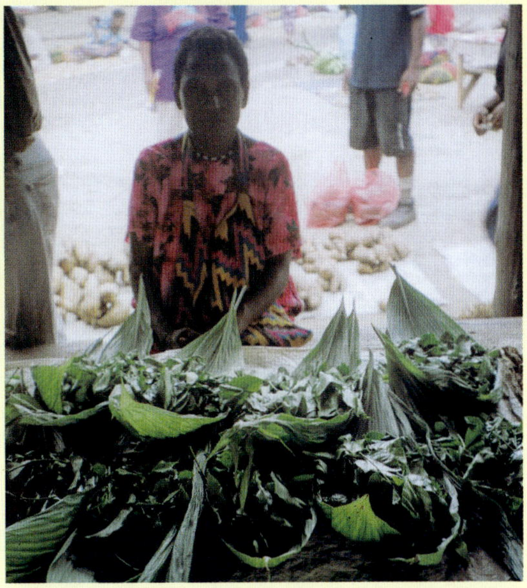

For you to try

- Write down some rules and customs related to food that you follow in your home or that other people follow.
- Explain why rules and customs related to food differ from one area to another.
- Write two rules or customs about food that you would like to follow or improve. Give reasons for your choice.

PLANNING MEALS USING LOCALLY AVAILABLE FOOD

When we prepare a meal for people to eat we want the food to be healthy. Healthy food is nutritious or **nourishing**. Meals that contain food from the three main food groups are usually nutritious, but other nutrients are also needed.

- Carbohydrates are needed for energy. There are two types—starches and sugar.
- Proteins are needed for growth of bones, skin, blood and muscles.
- Fats are needed to insulate the body from the cold, to protect organs and to provide energy.
- Minerals such as iron, phosphorus and calcium help the body to work properly.
- Vitamins are needed to protect the body against sickness.
- Fibre is needed to help move waste through the intestines.
- Water is needed for every body function. About three-quarters of the body is made of water.

We should all eat a balanced diet, but at certain times some people need to eat more of certain kinds of food.

- Children who are still growing need to eat plenty of protein food.
- Women who are pregnant need to eat plenty of protein, and food containing calcium (like milk) to help the baby to grow.
- People who are very active, do hard physical work or play sport need to eat more energy food.
- People who are sick need to eat more food to help them get better.
- People living in a cold place need to eat more energy food than people living in a hot place.
- People living in hot places need to drink plenty of liquids.

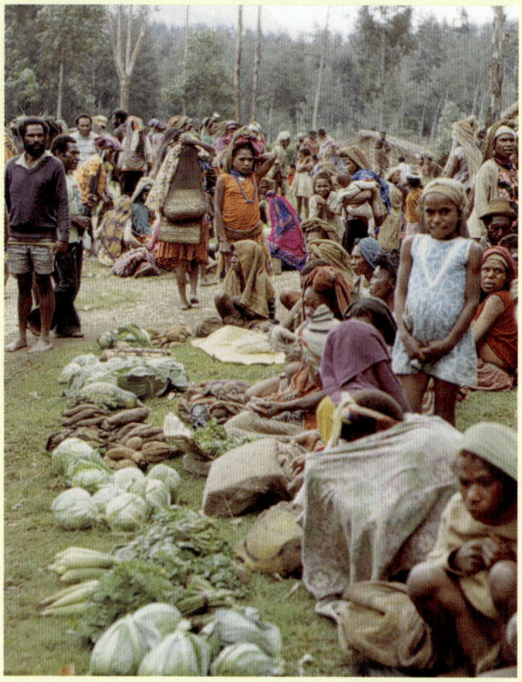

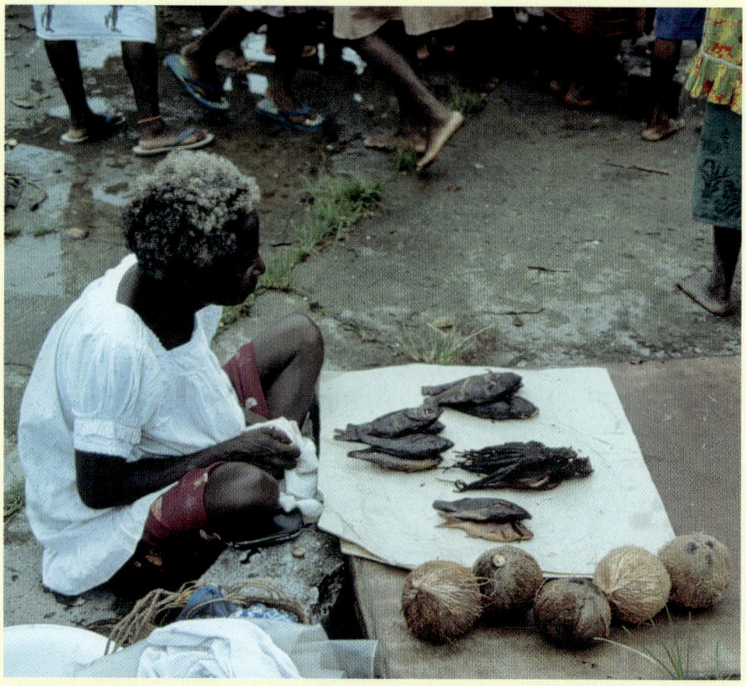

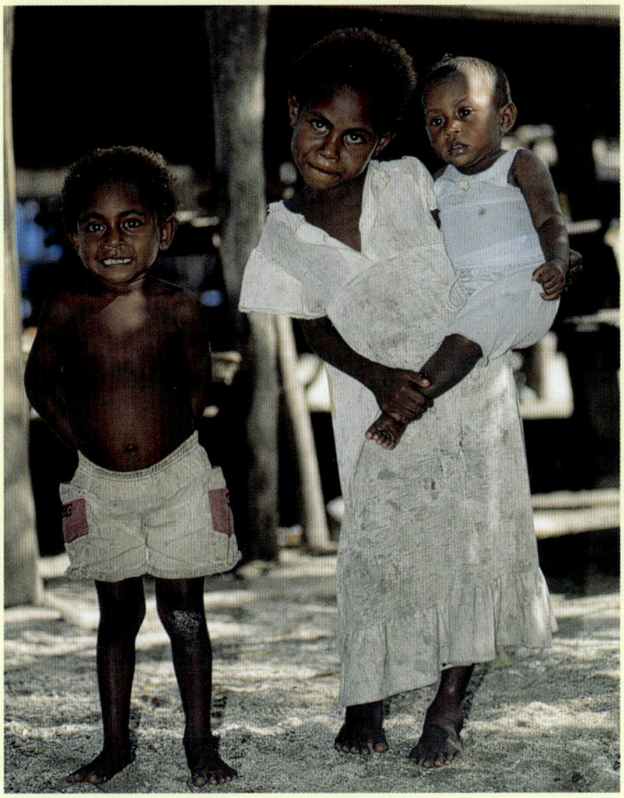

Growing children need to eat healthy food

For you to try

- Copy and complete the following table:

	Coastal food	Highlands food
Energy food that contains carbohydrates and fats		
Growth food that contains protein		
Protective food that contains vitamins and minerals		

- Make a poster to teach people about one of the following:
  — The importance of eating nutritious meals.
  — The importance of eating extra food for some groups of people (such as pregnant mothers or people who are very active).
- The class should divide into groups of four or five students. Each group should plan a simple meal that they can prepare at school. Each student should bring something that is needed to prepare the meal in the next class. After you have prepared the meal, share it with other groups. Which groups prepared nutritious meals? Explain why the meal was nutritious.

Personal health and safety

HEALTH CONCERNS

Newspapers often reflect the common health concerns of society. The extracts from newspaper articles below describe important issues such as domestic violence, drug abuse and HIV/AIDS.

Domestic violence not on

Women seeking hospital treatment after being beaten at home is becoming an import-ant reason for visiting the doctor, according to the Superintendent at the Provincial Hospital.

'We are seeing some women with quite serious injuries, especially after pay weekends,' he said.

Just recently one woman had to be flown to Port Moresby.

The Superintendent appealed to people not to ignore domestic violence when they know it is happening but to seek help from other family members and church leaders.

Drugs arrests

Four people have been charged for drugs offences following a tip-off to the police. The four were caught when they came to collect their cargo, which had been sent by air freight.

A local community leader has praised the public for providing information to the police which led to the arrests.

'If we all work together we can help to prevent the problem getting bigger. Too many young people are getting involved in marijuana,' he told our reporter.

HIV and AIDS increase

There has been another increase in the number of people with AIDS, according to a report produced by the Health Department.

'People must understand that they can avoid HIV by not having sex. Otherwise they can protect themselves from HIV by having only one faithful partner and by using condoms,' a health department spokesman said.

'We don't have to be afraid of people who are sick with AIDS, but we do have to be responsible in our personal relation-ships,' he told our reporter.

Drunk driver kills three

Three people were killed and several injured on the weekend following a fatal accident between two PMVs.

The accident happened on the Hiritano Highway. According to a police spokesman, both drivers had been drinking and passengers in the back of both vehicles were also drinking.

'Drinking and driving is very dangerous and it is also against the law for passengers to drink while travelling in any vehicle,' the police spokesman said.

HEALTH GOALS

Many of the things that we do in our lives will have an effect on our health. Some will help us to be healthy and some will make us unhealthy. We need to make healthy choices. Everyone can have health goals like the ones below:

- Take regular exercise and take part in leisure activities.
- Say 'no' to drugs.
- Be clean and hygienic in the way that you live.
- Avoid unsafe or dangerous situations.
- Have good relationships with other people.
- Develop positive self-esteem—feel good about yourself and the things that you can do.
- Learn how to deal with difficult and dangerous situations.

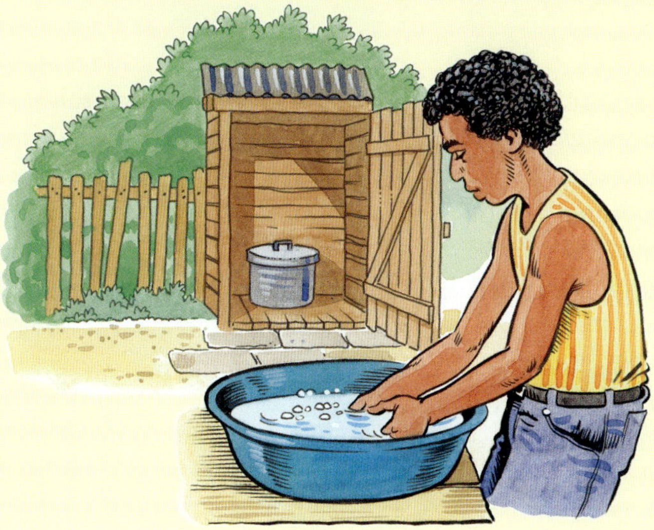

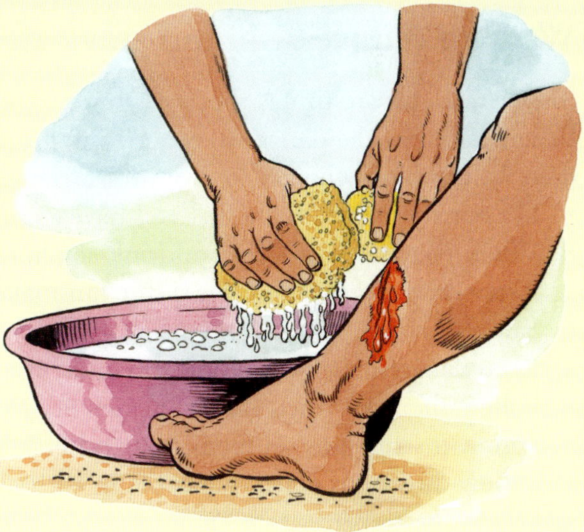

For you to try

- Write a letter that you could send to a newspaper about a health concern in the community, similar to those described in the four reports on page 42. Remember that newspapers usually like letters to be on a topic that will interest the readers. The letter should be short but make the main idea clear.
- What are the most important health concerns that affect your community?
- Choose a health goal like the ones mentioned above and develop a personal health plan that will help you to achieve this plan

RISKS

A **risk** is a behaviour that can have a bad effect on our health or wellbeing. There are many risks and hazards to our health and wellbeing at school, at home and in the community. We need to understand the link between our behaviour and its effect on our health. Some of these effects are described in the table below:

Behaviour	Effect on our health and other people
Smoking tobacco	Short of breath, lung diseases, cancer, bad smell
Drinking alcohol	Fighting, domestic violence, road accidents, short of money
Using marijuana	Spoils some parts of the brain, road accidents
Having unsafe sex	Sexually transmitted infections, HIV and AIDS, unwanted pregnancy, infertility (unable to become a mother or a father)

ML Ways to reduce risk and stay safe

S Safety measures are things that we can do in order to protect ourselves from harm and to stay healthy. When we know the danger that can come from the things that we do or that might happen to us, then we can make choices to avoid those dangers. For example:

- Do not start to smoke. Or if you have started smoking—stop.
- When you are old enough to drink alcohol, drink only a little.
- *Never* drink methylated spirits—it can make you go blind and may kill you.
- Say 'no' to drugs like marijuana.
- Keep dangerous objects and substances like kerosene and medicines away from children.
- Follow the rules when doing any activity that can be dangerous.
- Follow instructions on medicines and bottles of cleaning materials, and other signs.
- Follow directions given by people in authority like parents, teachers, police.
- Do not go to places that are unsafe.
- We need to show that we know and understand the danger by the way that we behave. Some people may think 'It will not happen to me', but risks can affect everyone.

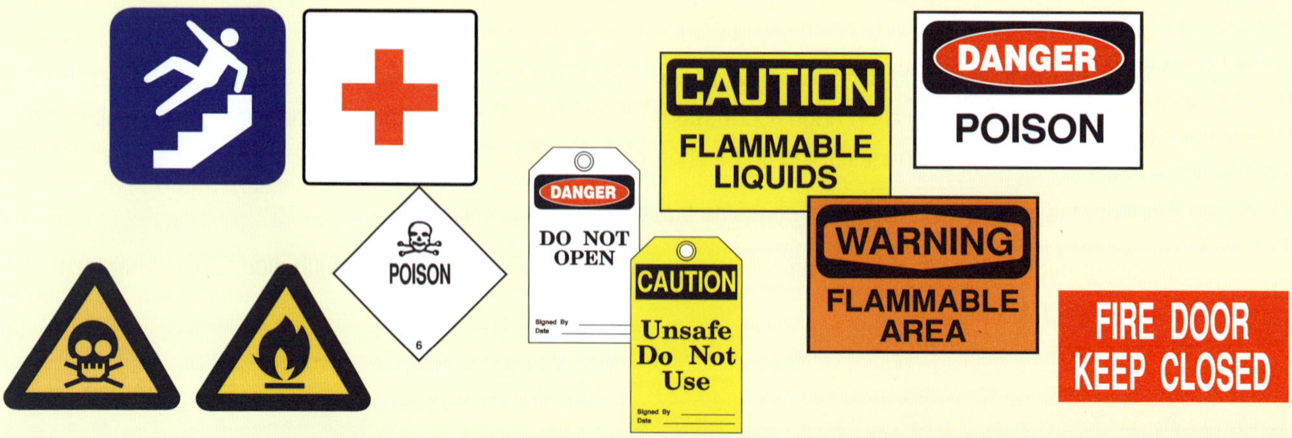
POISON
6
DANGER
DO NOT OPEN
CAUTION
FLAMMABLE LIQUIDS
CAUTION
Unsafe Do Not Use
DANGER
POISON
WARNING
FLAMMABLE AREA
FIRE DOOR KEEP CLOSED

These signs warn us about dangers and help us stay safe.

For you to try

- Make a list of dangerous objects and substances and say how you would protect children against these.
- Make a list of things that you can do at home and at school in order to stay safe.
- Make a plan for what you would do if you found yourself in a dangerous situation. How do you know when it is not safe? What can you do to make yourself safe again?

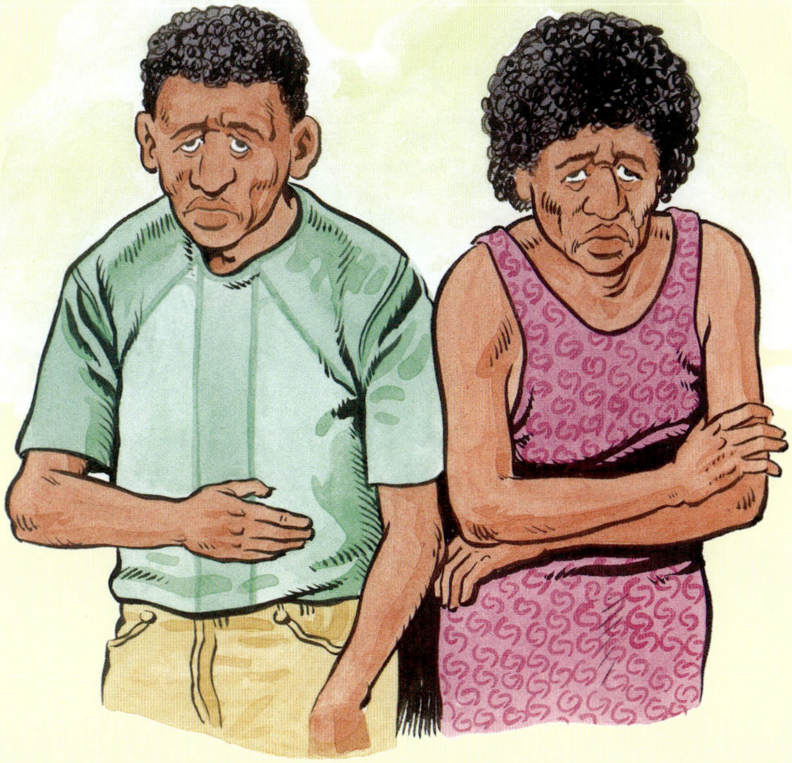

Alcohol has many bad effects on our health

Behaviour that affects our safety

Sometimes people behave in ways that can affect the safety of other people and that can spoil the surroundings. Some *causes* are:

- drinking in public places like sports ovals, near shops or in the market
- drinking and driving
- throwing rubbish like bottles
- smoking in public places like buildings
- chewing and spitting betel nut
- writing on walls—graffiti
- making trouble for other people for no good reason
- rape.

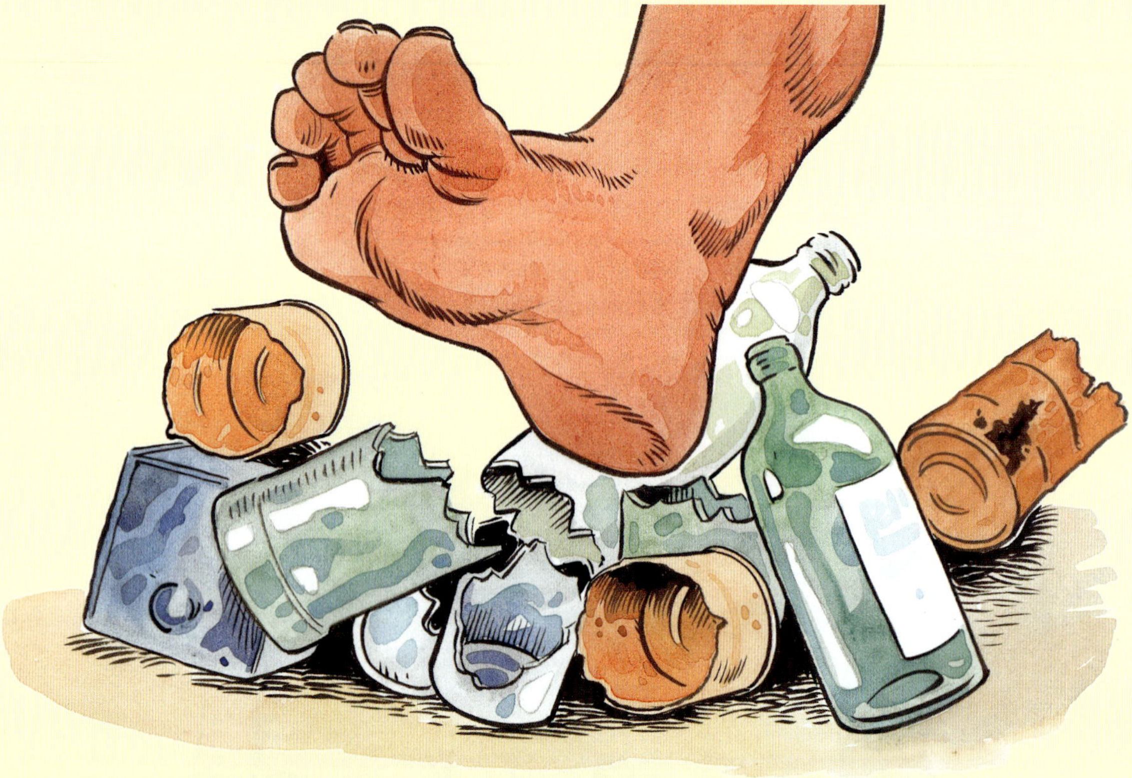

These types of behaviour can have various *effects* on other people and the places where we all live. For example:

- fighting
- accidents and even death
- damage to property
- damage to the environment
- sexually transmitted infections (also known as sexually transmitted diseases)
- unwanted pregnancy.

For you to try

- Choose some examples of causes of behaviour from the list above and make some links with the effects of the behaviour.
- Write two or three paragraphs on how we can reduce the causes of behaviour that have a negative effect on the lives of people in the community.
- Do one of the following:
  — Design a poster to tell people about healthy and positive living. Display your poster in the community.
  — Make up a short play about healthy and positive living. Practise your play and show it to the rest of your class and to the community.

Community health

HEALTH PROMOTION ML

There are many things that we can do in order take care of our health. These are choices that we make in order to be healthy. Choosing some behaviour and not others is the main way that we can stay healthy.

Health workers say that *prevention is better than cure*. This means that it is better to try to stop sickness before it happens than to wait until people are sick and then try to make them better. However, if you do get sick, it is important to get treatment quickly and not wait until you get worse.

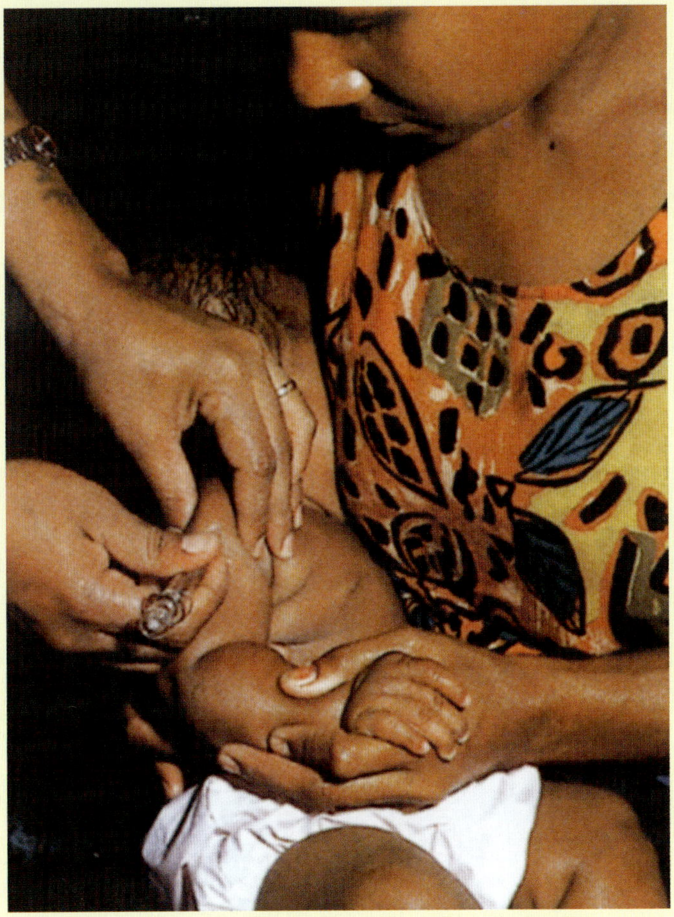

Immunisation protects children against common illnesses

All of the things that we do in order to prevent or reduce sickness and to stay healthy are called **health promotion.** For example:

- Health education—teaching people to find out about the causes of sickness and how to stay healthy so that they know what to do. This is done by the government, churches, in newspapers, on the radio and television.
- Immunisation—giving injections or vaccinations to children as they grow up in order to protect them against illnesses that are common in children. Mothers can also be given vaccinations to help prevent sickness.

- A clean and reliable water supply that provides safe water for drinking and cooking, as well as for washing.
- Toilets that are used properly and kept clean. All kinds of toilets can be healthy if they are made and used properly.
- A way to get rid of rubbish that prevents flies and rats and does not spoil the surroundings.
- Eating a balanced diet or eating the right amount of different kinds of food every day.

Recommended immunisation program in Papua New Guinea

Age	Vaccination
Soon after birth	BCG
2 months	Triple antigen and Sabin (in town)
4 months	Triple antigen and Sabin (in town)
6 months	Triple antigen and Sabin (in town)
7 years	BCG and tetanus toxoid
13 years	BCG and tetanus toxoid
First baby (for mothers)	Tetanus toxoid
Fourth baby (for mothers)	Tetanus toxoid

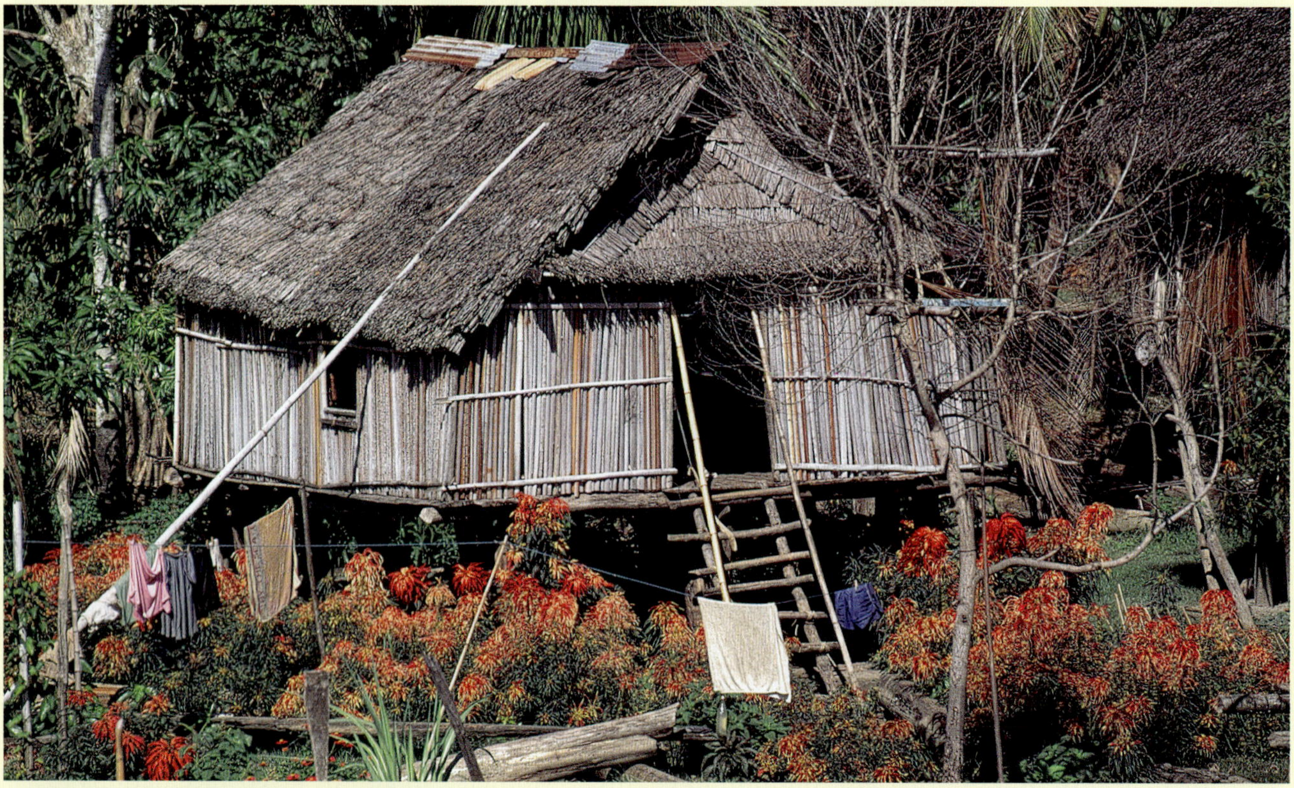

A healthy, clean environment is important

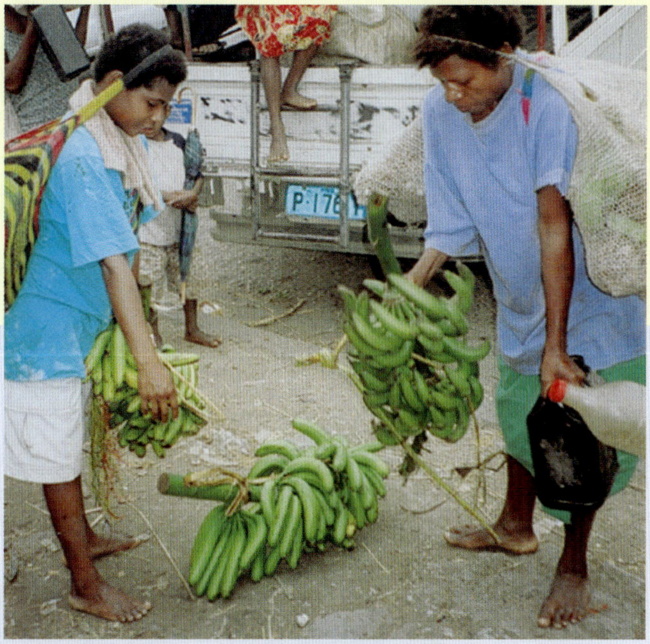

Fruit is part of a balanced diet

For you to try

- What are the traditional and modern ways of living a healthy way of life in your area? Discuss as a group and write down your ideas.
- Carry out a survey to find out what immunisations or vaccination the students in your class have received. Use the following table, and make a bar chart to show your results.

Recommended immunisation program in Papua New Guinea

	Age				
Immunisation or vaccination	**1st**	**2nd**	**3rd**	**4th / 5th**	**Number of students who have completed this vaccination**
BCG for tuberculosis	Birth	Age 3	Age 13		
Hepatitis B	Birth	1 month	3 months		
Triple antigen for diphtheria, whooping cough and tetanus	1 month	2 months	3 months		
Sabin for polio	Birth	1 month	2 months	3 months	
Pigbel	1 month	2 months	3 months	7 and 13 years	
Measles	6 months	9 months			
Tetanus toxoid for tetanus	7 years	3 years			

- Look for messages about health promotion or health education in and around your community. Look for posters, pamphlets, newspaper articles or advertisements on the radio and television. What is the main message? What is the behaviour that people have to follow in order to stay healthy?
- Choose an illness that is common in your area or another part of Papua New Guinea. What health promotion activities can we use in order to teach people how to prevent or reduce this health problem?

THE ENVIRONMENT AND HEALTH

For thousands of years people in Papua New Guinea lived in small communities, grew their own food and went hunting and fishing. This way of life is sometimes called **subsistence agriculture**. People used their traditional knowledge, and their way of life did not spoil the environment. There was enough fresh water and firewood and the waste that they produced did not cause problems. This can be a very healthy way to live. Some people in PNG are still living in this way.

When a country is developing, people start to live in towns and cities and the way of life begins to change. There is not enough land for every family to grow food, so people must buy food. People then need to earn money to be able to buy food. Getting enough fresh water and firewood and getting rid of waste can also become a problem when a lot of people live close together.

Towns and cities also have factories for making goods, and these factories also produce waste that can spoil the environment. Mining and logging in rural areas can cause the same sort of problem. For example, waste products from factories and mines may run into rivers and creeks, making the water unfit to drink and killing the fish.

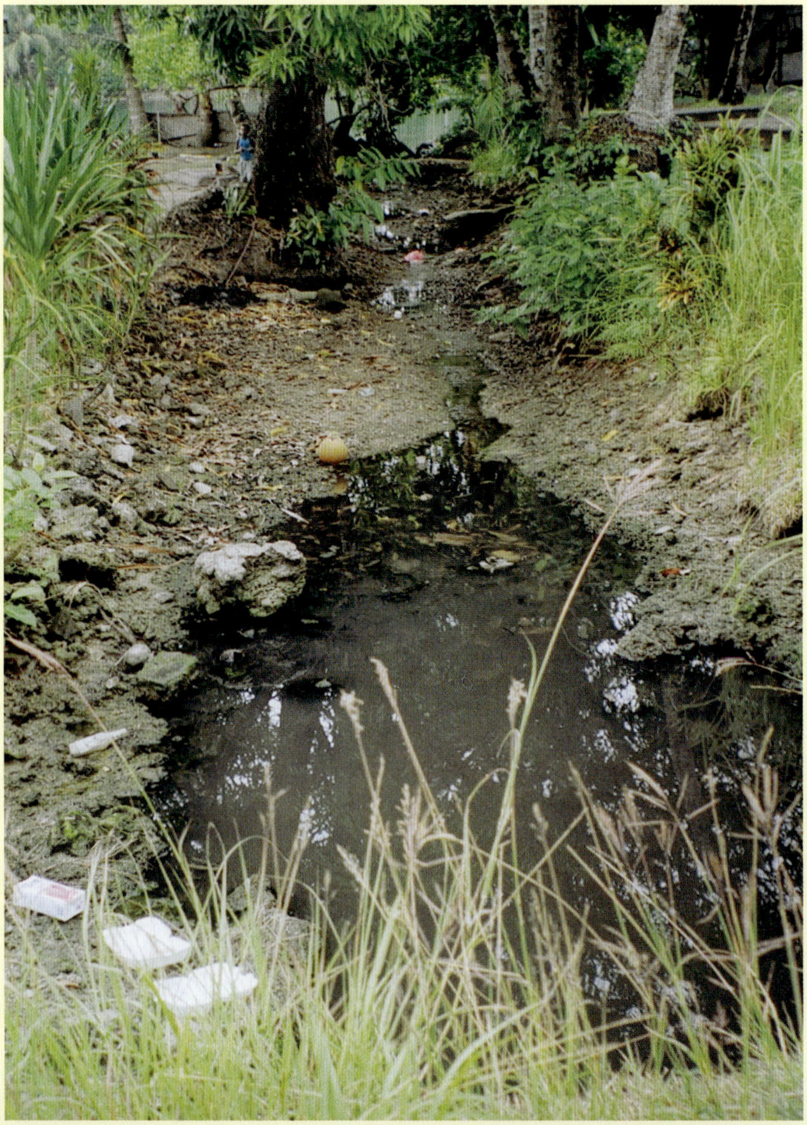

The dirty water will eventually run into the sea where it can still affect people. Towns and cities also have many cars and trucks and the exhaust can make the air dirty, especially in big cities.

The way that waste products from towns, cities and other developments can change and spoil the surroundings is called **pollution**. Pollution can affect the land, rivers, sea and air. Pollution is important because it can have a negative effect on the health of people. Pollution can also be carried big distances, so the people who are affected may be living a long way from the place where the pollution started—even in a different country.

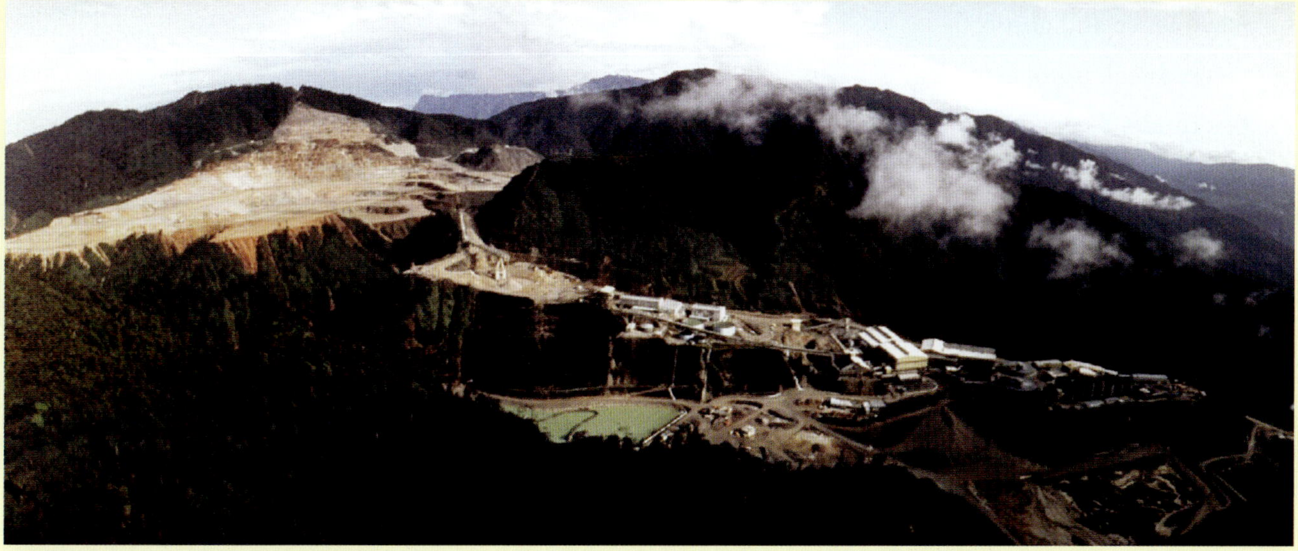

Some mining activities cause pollution

EFFECTS OF DEVELOPMENT ON HEALTH

The things that we do as part of development can have an effect on our health. For example:

- We can spoil rivers and creeks used for drinking and fishing. We can also spoil the sea, killing fish or killing reefs.
- We can destroy areas used for hunting, gardening and harvesting traditional medicine. For example, cutting down forests can mean that soil is washed away during heavy rain.
- People can get sick from dirty water and air, as well as from land that is polluted. For example, people may get diarrhoea or gastroenteritis.
- Some mines, factories and plantations use chemicals that can make people sick. These chemicals can get into the water supply.

For you to try

- Find out about and describe some changes in the environment caused by the activities of people in Papua New Guinea. What are the causes and effects of the changes on the health of people and other living things? You can choose some small changes in your area or a big project like a mine, a timber project or a plantation.
- A Carry out a survey to look at the environment of your school or community. Make a plan to improve this environment.

The use of drugs

The use of tobacco, alcohol and other drugs like marijuana is becoming a big problem in Papua New Guinea. Tobacco and alcohol are both having a big effect on the health of people. Some of the negative effects of these drugs are:

- diseases like lung disease and liver disease
- accidents and deaths like road accidents
- violence and abuse
- the break up of families
- crime.

REASONS WHY PEOPLE CHOOSE TO TAKE DRUGS

There are many reasons why people smoke cigarettes, drink beer, wine and spirits or take other drugs. For example:

- the way that they feel about themselves—their thoughts and feelings
- the way that they are affected by their parents, family and friends
- the way that they are affected by other people in the community
- the way that they are affected by the media—newspapers, radio and television.

Many young people start to smoke and drink because smoking and drinking are things that adults do and young people want others to see them as grown up. Unfortunately, tobacco contains a drug called **nicotine** which is **addictive**. This means that once people start to smoke they find it very hard to stop, even though they may know that smoking can make them sick. Many smokers started when they were young and wanted to act like adults, but now they wish that they had never started. In countries like Australia, young people under the age of eighteen are not allowed to buy cigarettes or alcohol.

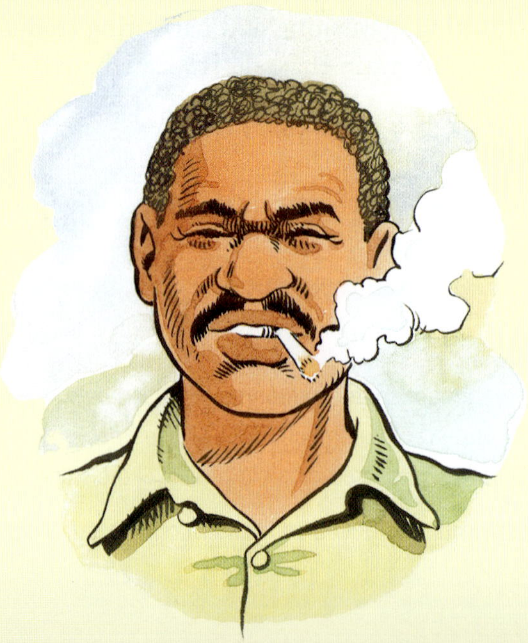

THE EFFECTS OF SMOKING, ALCOHOL AND OTHER DRUGS

When people smoke tobacco they can get a number of diseases, including lung diseases like lung cancer. Tobacco smoke can also affect other people who breathe in the smoke, even when they are not smoking. This is called **passive smoking.** Smoking causes more sickness in the world than any other reason, so if people stop smoking a lot of sickness will be prevented.

In Papua New Guinea smoking is also not allowed in public buildings or on aeroplanes. In many countries in the world cigarettes have a warning on the packet telling people that smoking can damage their health.

Beer, wine and spirits all contain alcohol, which can help people to relax on social occasions. Wine is also used in some religious ceremonies. For example, in some churches, a small amount of wine is drunk during communion.

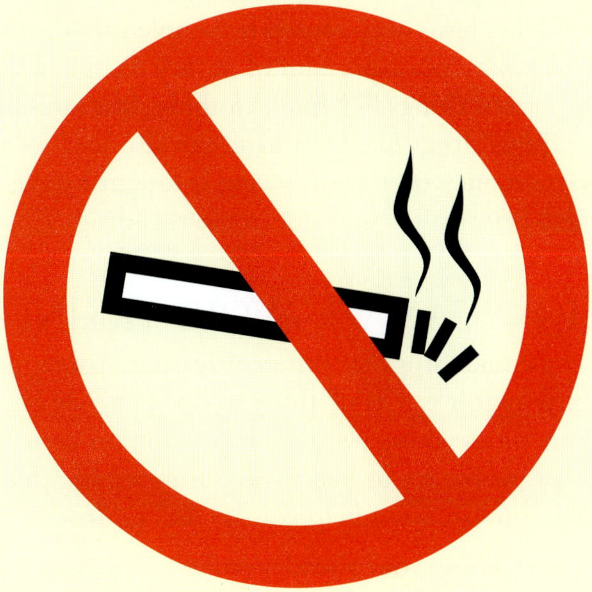

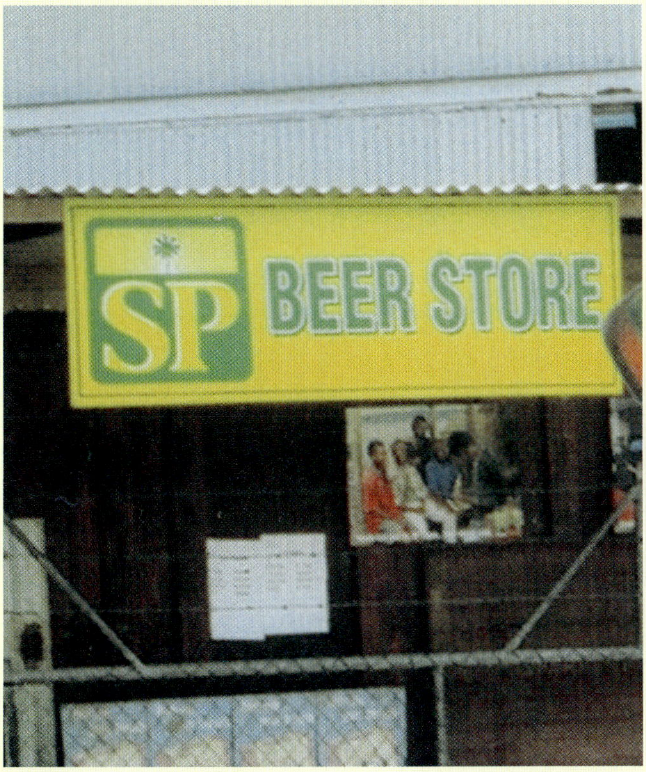

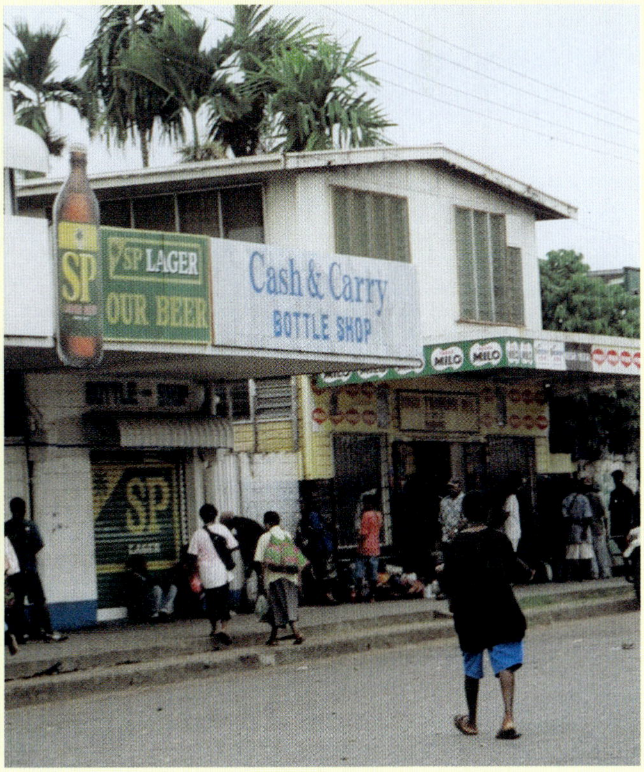

When people drink a lot of alcohol, it begins to affect the brain and the way that people behave. For example, people can no longer think properly and they may fall over or start to fight and hurt other people and damage property. People who have been drinking should not drive. Many road accidents have been caused by people driving after they have been drinking.

Alcohol also costs a lot of money. People who drink a lot may not have enough money for more important things like food, clothing, bus fares and school fees.

Illegal drugs like marijuana can also lead to diseases of the lungs and mental illness. People can waste money on this drug, and if caught by the police they may be convicted and sent to prison. For these reasons it is best not to use this drug.

HOW CAN WE AVOID TAKING DRUGS?

People take drugs for different reasons. Young people often start to smoke or to drink because they think that it is a 'cool' thing to do. They see adults doing these things and they want to act like adults. Sometimes young people put pressure on their friends to try out new things. What can you do when other people try to make you do something that you don't want to do? There are a number of things that you can do to help you say 'no' to drugs:

- Choose your friends carefully. Other people who take drugs may want you to take them or you may feel like following them.
- Learn to make up your own mind and to follow your own thinking. Do not follow other people when they are doing something illegal or harmful.

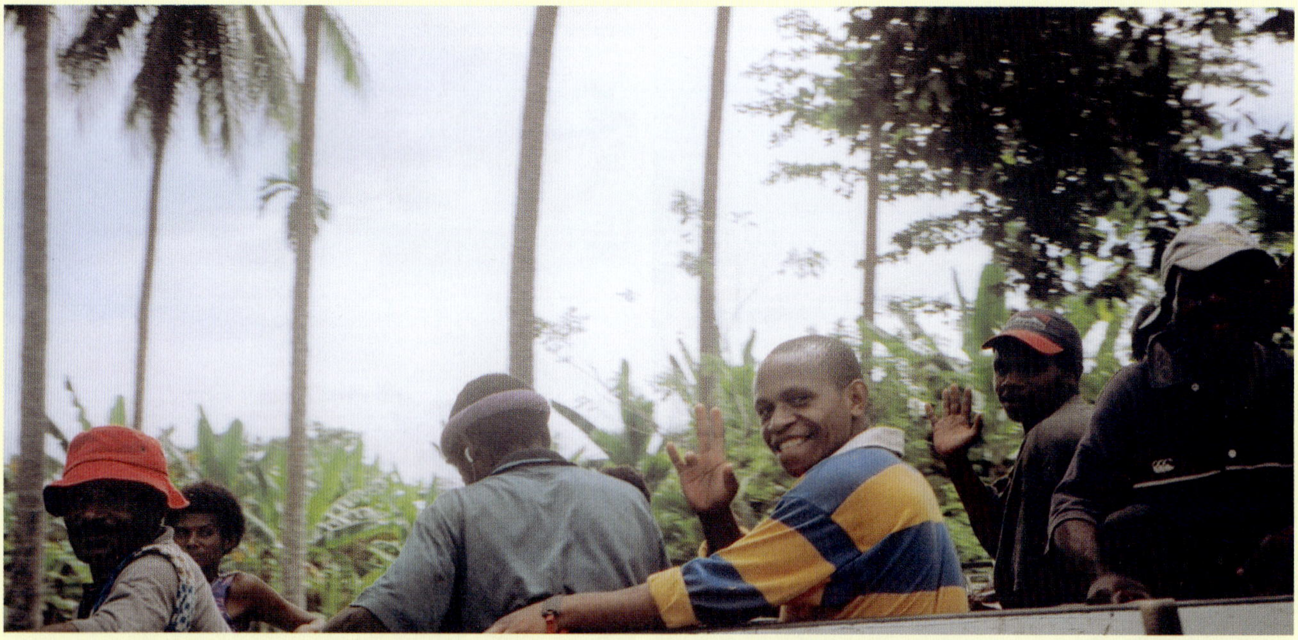

- If people try to force you, just smile and tell them that you have already thought about it and made up your mind that you don't want to take drugs.
- If people are doing something that is against the law or that is harmful, do not stay with them. Go somewhere else.
- Take part in other activities like sports, youth groups and church groups.
- If you decide to drink when you are old enough, then drink only a little. Do not get drunk. Do not drive after drinking.

For you to try

- Copy and complete the following:

Smoking cigarettes or tobacco

Positive effects	Negative effects

Draw similar tables for other drugs like alcohol and marijuana.

- Describe the effects of the decisions that people make about taking drugs on the health of the person who takes the drug and on the community.
- In pairs or in small groups, discuss the feelings, thoughts and attitudes of you and your family about people who take drugs.

For you to try

- In pairs, role play and practise different ways of saying 'no' to drugs.
- Find out the names of people and organisations that can help people to stop taking drugs.
- Imagine that you have a friend who has a problem with drugs. What would you do in order to help?

5

Living and Working Together

Chapter Summary

In this chapter you will have an opportunity to:

- ✔ Find out about taking part in the community and helping other people
- ✔ Find out about the positive and negative effects of the choices that we make
- ✔ Find out about the work of leaders in a community
- ✔ Find out about the reasons for laws and the way that they help people
- ✔ Describe what might happen if people lose their rights and freedoms

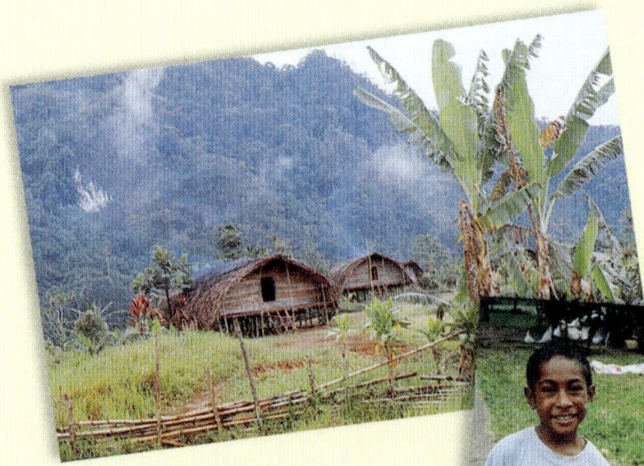

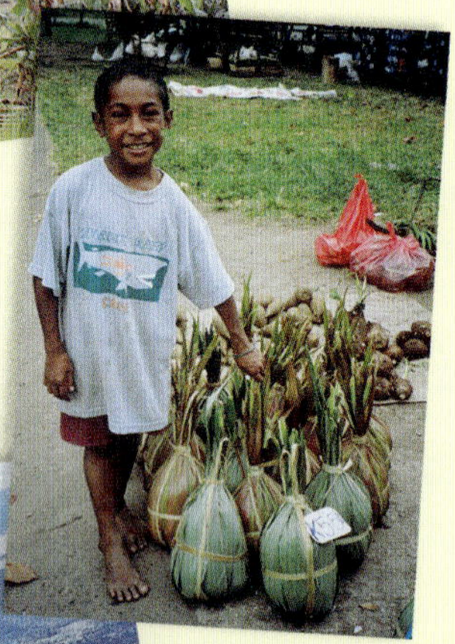

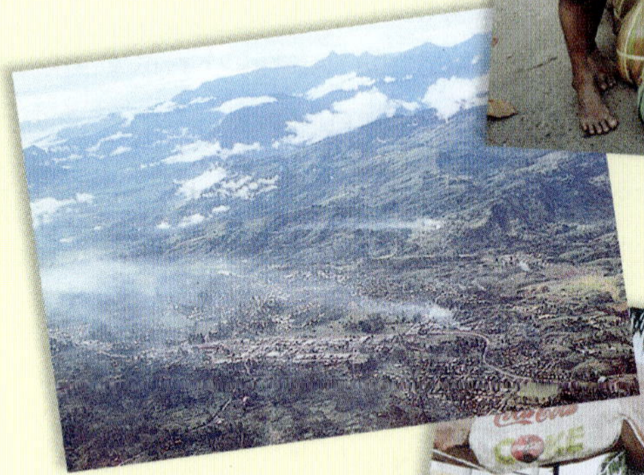

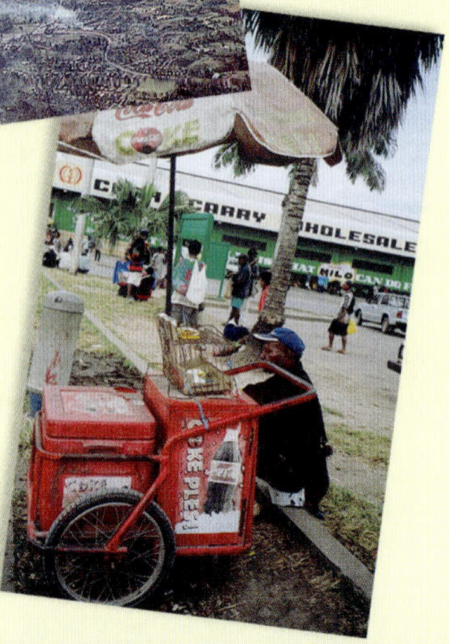

Syllabus references

Strand: Living and working together
Sub-strands: Making choices, good and fair leaders, rule of law, respecting rights and freedoms

Outcomes:

7.5.1 Describe how participating in community service helps the whole community

7.5.2 Outline the positive and negative results of making choices

7.5.3 Explain the roles and responsibilities of leaders in a community

7.5.4 Explain the purpose and benefits of laws in our society

7.5.5 Explain what could happen if the rights and freedom of people are violated or abused

Making choices

REASONS FOR TAKING PART IN THE COMMUNITY ML

Key facts

- When we take an active part in the community in which we live, we help everyone else in the community.
- When we make choices there can be both positive and negative results which come from those choices. Some choices may affect only ourselves and other choices will affect others in the community.
- Leaders in the community have particular roles and responsibilities, and the community has expectations about the way that leaders carry out their roles.
- Rules and laws are needed to give people the right and freedom to live safely and be protected against other people.
- If rights and freedoms are taken away, then people will be afraid and will not be able to live safely together.

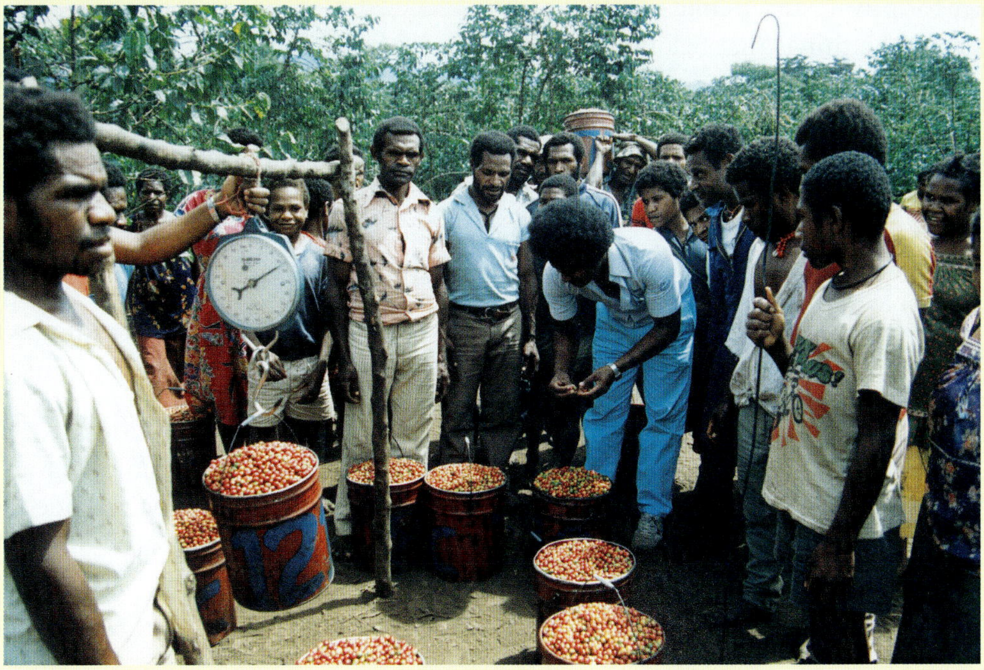

When we live together in a community there are many things that need to be done in order to help the community. For example, we need to keep the place clean and tidy and everyone can help to do this by getting rid of rubbish. From time to time we all need help with the things that we do and so we should also be ready to help other people when they need help. If you are willing to give help to other people, then they will be more likely to give help to you and to others when it is needed. When people help each other in this way, and when they know and respect each other, they will also be able to sort out problems in the community when they occur.

The way that people look after a community and the way that they treat each other tells us a lot about the community.

ML VALUES WE USE TO HELP MAKE DECISIONS

The **values** that people have are the things that they say or think are important. Values come from the things that people believe are good and right and true. We all begin to learn values when we are children and we continue throughout our lives. Parents and teachers help children to develop the values that are accepted in the community. We also learn values from being a member of a church or a religion and from other groups in the community.

We show our values by the way that we behave, not just by what we say. The values that we use to make decisions are shown below:

Respect

- respect for myself and others
- respect for laws and for authority
- respect for private and public property—the things that belong to other people and the community

Honesty

- being fair and trustworthy
- being reliable and dependable
- knowing and admitting when other people are dishonest

Obligations—things that you must do

- obligations to your family and community
- being open-minded, ready to listen, not too quick to judge other people
- being interested in the community and prepared to ask questions

Concern

- being kind and considerate and understanding the feelings of other people
- being cooperative and accepting that people are different and that there can be more than one way of doing things
- sharing in decision-making

Dedication

- knowing and understanding what is happening in the community
- taking part in community activities
- helping the community before helping yourself—being civic-minded

Justice

- being fair and treating people equally
- respecting the rights of other people
- letting the law do the job that it has to do

For you to try

- Describe some things that have been done in the community where you live or another community that you know. What values are associated with these activities?
- Carry out a survey to find out the needs of your community. Suggest ways that the community could meet those needs.

People taking part in community activities

For you to try

- Describe some things that have been done in the community where you live or another community that you know. What values are associated with these activities?
- Carry out a survey to find out the needs of your community. Suggest ways that the community could meet those needs.

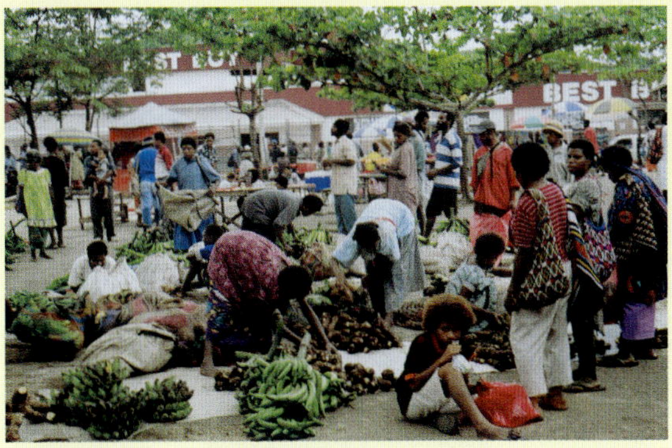

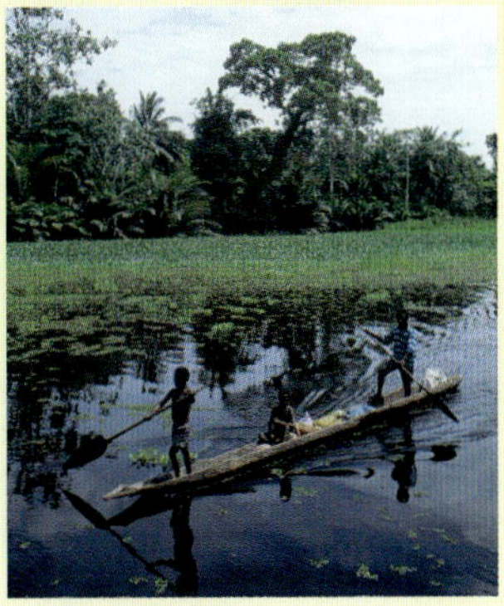

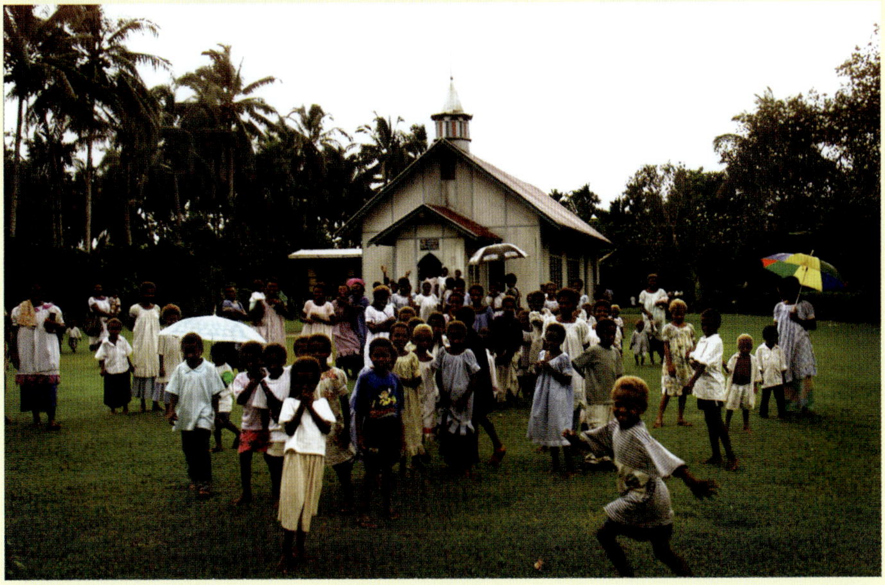

THE CHOICES THAT WE MAKE

When we are babies we cannot make any choices. The adults who take care of us make all these choices for us. As we grow up we all need to make choices every day of our lives.

Most people enjoy being able to make different choices. Some of these choices may be simple personal choices like what to eat and what to wear, but as we become adults, we learn to make more important choices about what to do. Some of these choices can be difficult to make and some can also be important to the community.

Some examples of personal choices are:

- to develop good relationships with friends and family
- to eat properly and to exercise regularly
- whether to smoke
- whether to drink alcohol
- whether to take drugs
- to decide what you will do when you leave school
- to decide if you want to get married and when to have sex

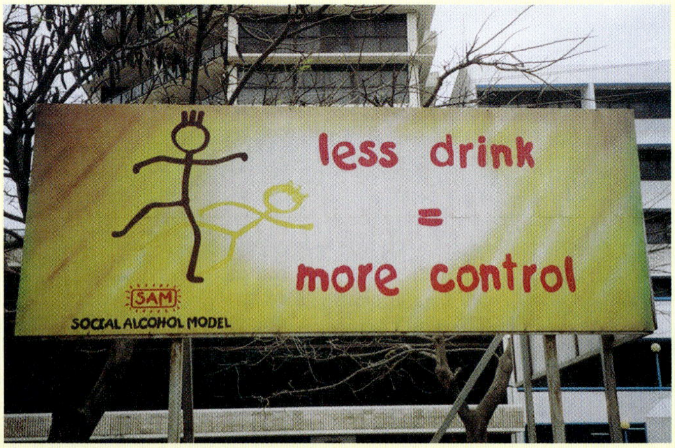

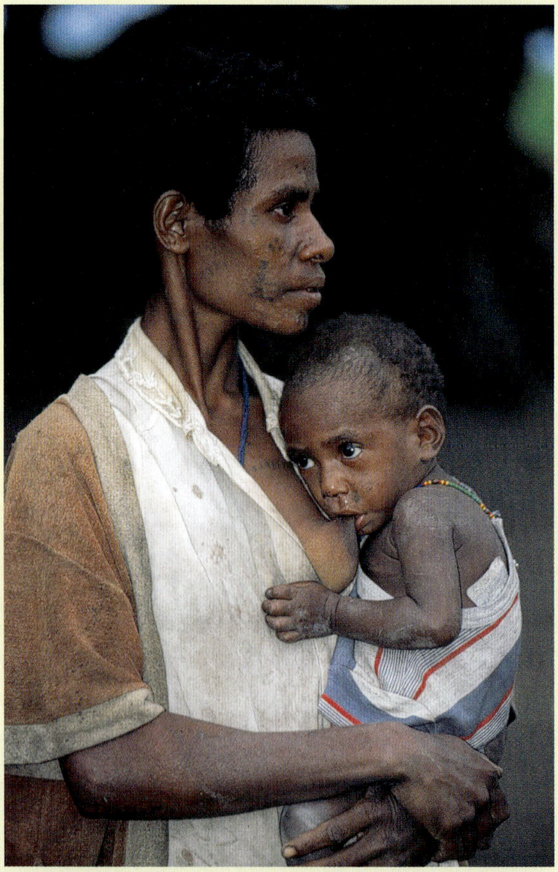

This mother makes important choices for her baby

Some examples of choices that can be important to the community are:

- to take part in community activities
- to take a position of leadership in the community
- to help to solve conflicts
- whether to sell cigarettes, alcohol or other drugs
- whether to take part in gambling

RESULTS OF THE CHOICES THAT WE MAKE

When we make a choice, things will happen as a result of that choice. Some of these results may be positive and some may be negative, so we think about the result before we make the choice. For example, when we eat properly and take exercise, then this will help us to be healthy. When we learn to give and take, then we will have better relationships with our family and friends. When we get rid of rubbish in the right place, then we help to keep the surroundings clean and healthy. These are all examples of the positive results of the choices that we make.

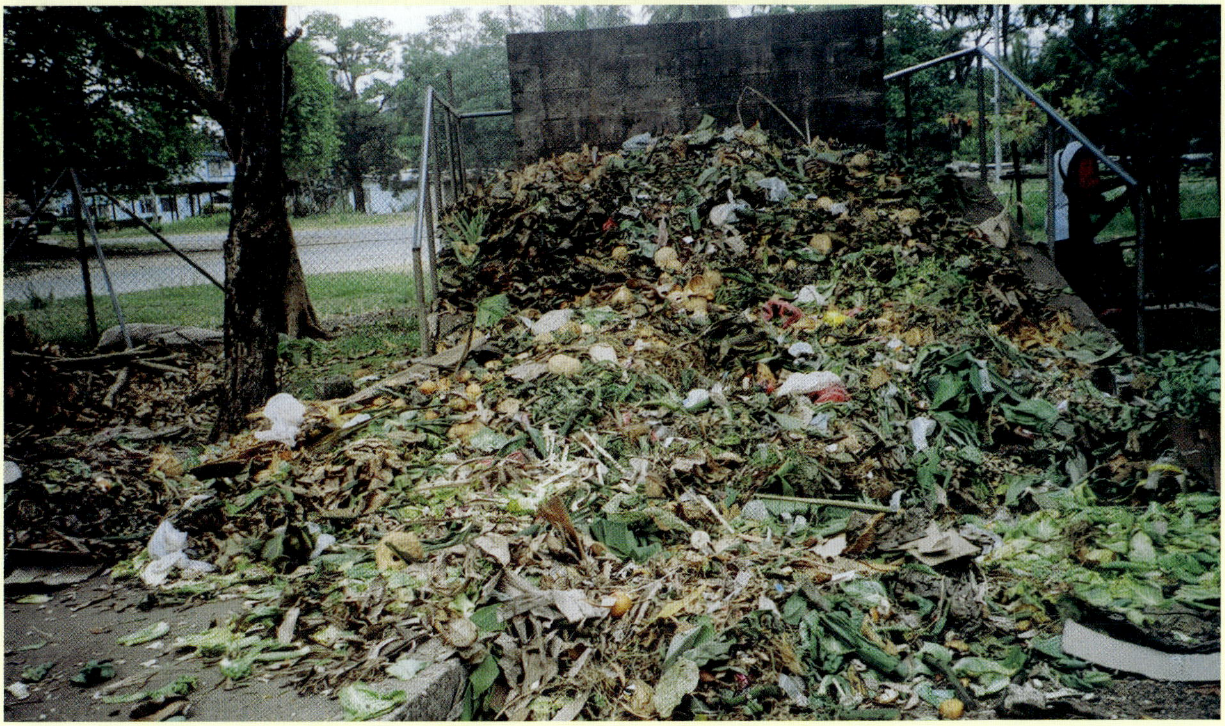

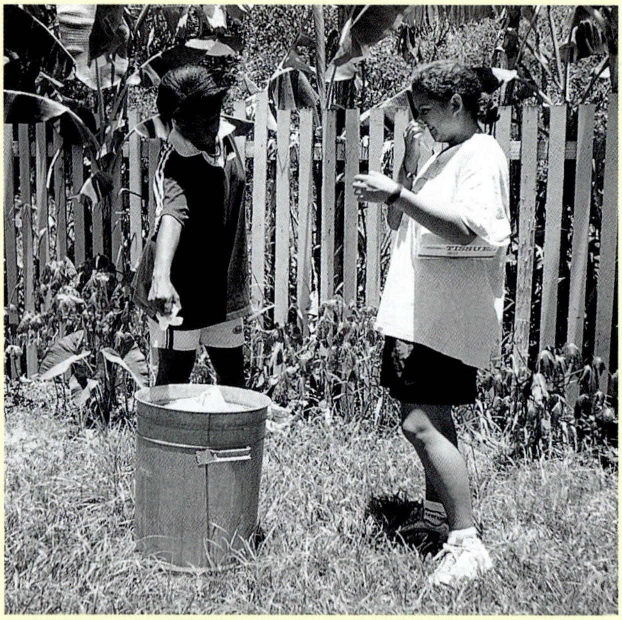

Sometimes there may be negative results from the choices that we make. For example, if we eat too many sweet foods and lolly water, then we may get tooth decay. If we gamble by playing cards we can lose a lot of money, and this can lead to other problems in the family. When we drink too much alcohol or take drugs, then this can lead to fighting and sickness. And when we have sex before we are ready, then this can lead to unwanted babies and to sexually transmitted infections.

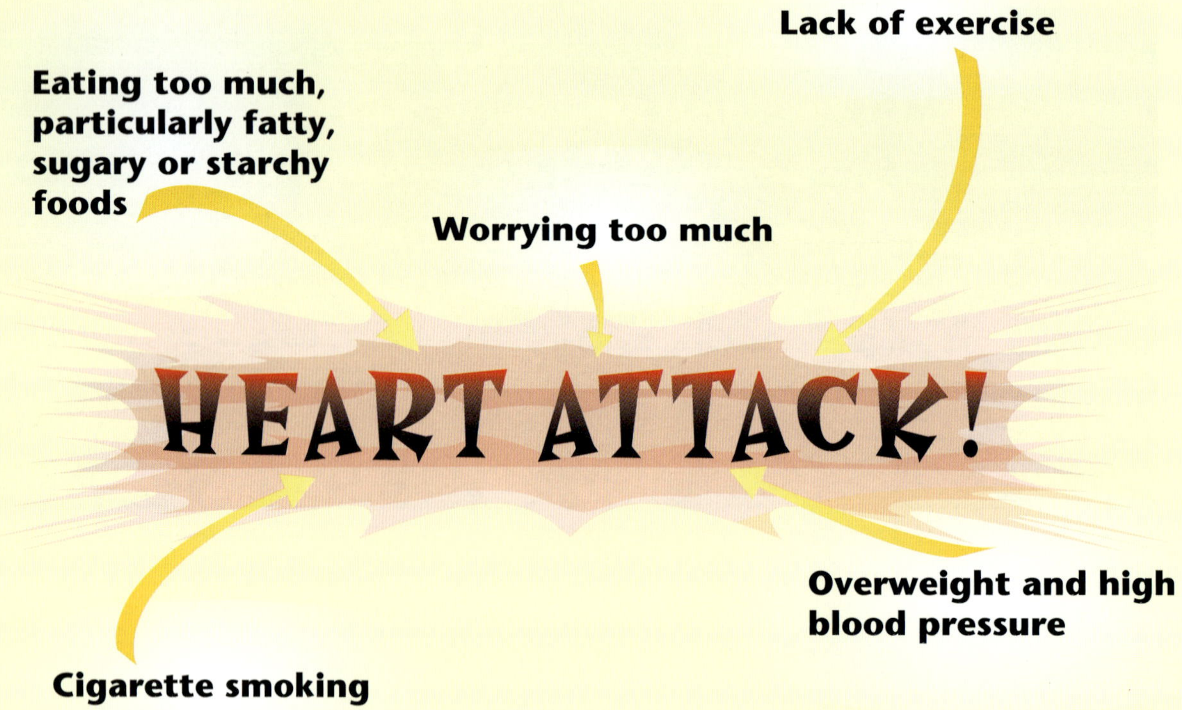

Good and fair leaders

WHAT SHOULD LEADERS DO? ML

When we choose our leaders it is their job to represent us and speak and act for all of us. We expect leaders to behave in certain ways, so being a good and fair leader is not always easy. We should respect leaders, but leaders also need to behave in ways which earn the respect of the people. Leaders should not expect other people to follow them just because they are leaders.

Things that we expect good leaders to do:

- Be responsible and ready to answer for the way that they behave.
- Represent the people in the community equally.
- Be open and honest in dealing with other people.
- Have a high standard of personal behaviour.
- Communicate openly with the community.
- Understand the needs and rights of everyone in the community.
- Listen to the community and to what other leaders say.
- Respect the community.

The **Leadership Code**, which is part of the Constitution, is a set of rules for Members of Parliament and senior public servants to follow so that they are honest and fair. The **Ombudsman Commission** makes sure that the Leadership Code is followed. Any person who believes that a leader is being dishonest or unfair can complain to the Ombudsman Commission, which will investigate the complaint and take action where necessary. A leader who is taken to court and convicted of an offence in relation to his position, or who does not follow the Leadership Code, is guilty of misconduct in office.

Leadership Code

Leaders should

- be unselfish and not allowed to be in a position where they can make decisions that will help themselves
- not behave in such a way that people do not respect them as people, the position they hold or the government in Papua New Guinea
- be honest and not try to help themselves because of their position as leaders
- make sure that their families and others who work for them behave in ways that show that the leader is following this code
- if necessary, make it clear to the public that they have not done anything wrong

For you to try

- Think about leaders in your school or your community. Discuss the things that they can do to help to improve the community.
- Describe the roles and responsibilities of leaders and members of the community.
- Write down some of the ways that leaders and community members can communicate in order to help the community and to keep the community healthy and peaceful.
- List five outstanding leaders from Papua New Guinea. Choose one as your personal role model and explain why you chose this person. Include a description of their qualities and achievements and the influence that they have had on other people.

ML Rules and laws

WHY WE HAVE LAWS

All communities have rules and laws which show people the way that they should behave and make it easier for people to live together in the community. There should always be a reason for having a rule or law and the reason should be clear to all people. When people understand the reason for the rule or the law, they are more likely to follow it.

Some reasons for having laws are:

- for safety and protection
- to be fair to everyone in the community, so that everyone is treated the same
- to protect the rights of individuals
- to maintain law and order in the community
- to help people to respect public property like schools, churches and playing fields
- to help people to live and work in peace
- to protect our resources, like plants and animals, the land and the environment

MAKING AND BREAKING RULES AND LAWS

The laws of Papua New Guinea are made by the national government or parliament and are the same for everybody in the country. Each province also has the power to make some of its own rules. For example, each province can make rules about the sale of alcohol. When there is fighting in a province, the sale of alcohol can be stopped until the fighting has stopped and the trouble is finished. Some local councils also make rules.

Many families have rules for family members. For example, some families have rules about the things that children can do and about sharing the jobs that need to be done, like helping to clean around the house.

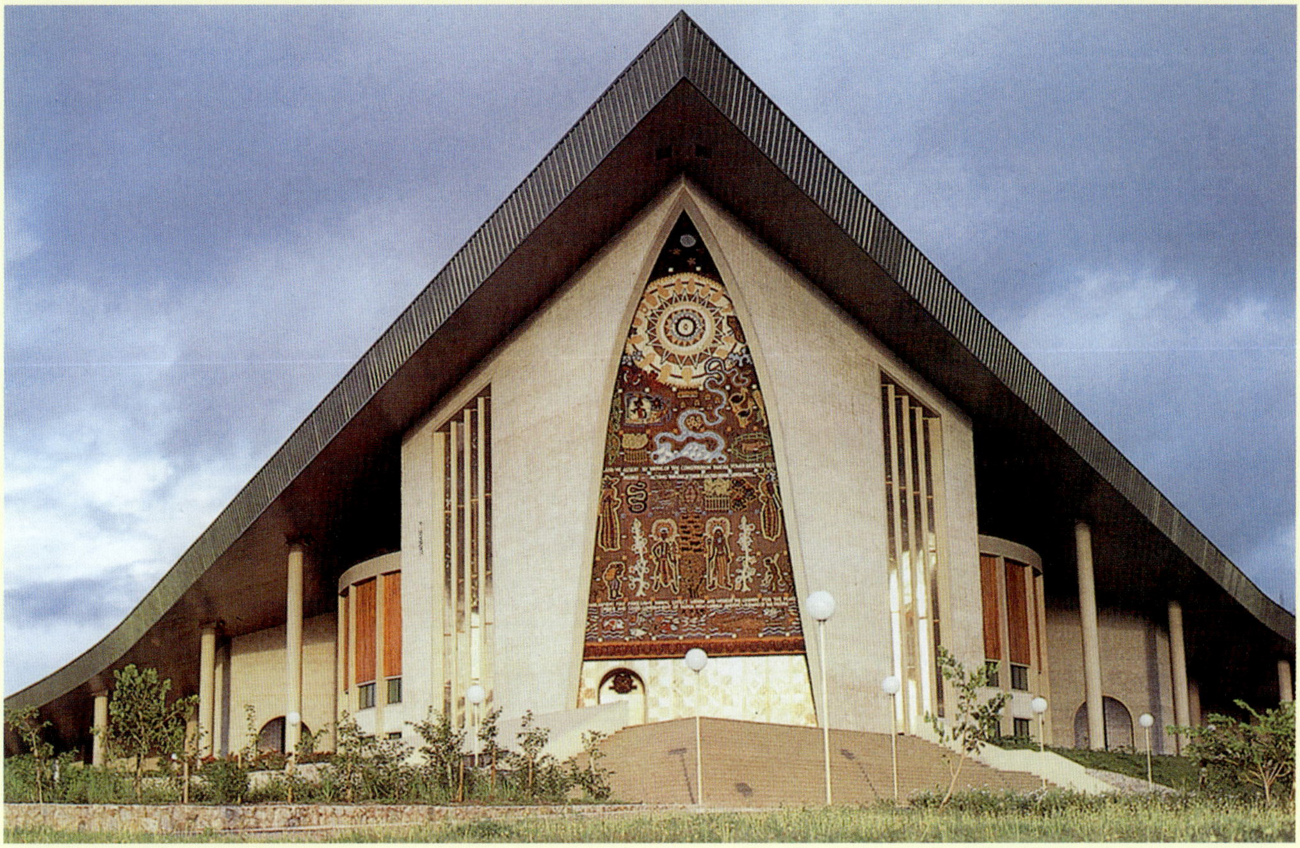

Parliament House, Port Moresby

Many people help to make sure that we follow rules and laws. For example:

- police
- army
- courts such as the Local Court, District Court and National Court
- community elders and councillors
- parents and teachers

When people follow the rules or laws, then there may be *rewards* to encourage people to continue to follow them. When people are caught breaking a rule or a law, then there is usually some sort of *punishment* which is intended to stop the person from breaking the rule or law in the future. If the police catch people who are breaking the law, they can take those people to court and the court may give the punishment. One form of punishment is to be sent to a Corrective Institution, like the one at Bomana outside Port Moresby. People do not like to be punished, so the punishment is a way of telling everybody not to break the law.

Rules and laws should be based on common sense—the things that most people believe to be fair or true. People who are experienced in making rules understand that it is better to keep them short and simple rather than to have long lists of rules for people to follow. The people who make rules should look at them regularly and remove those rules that are no longer needed.

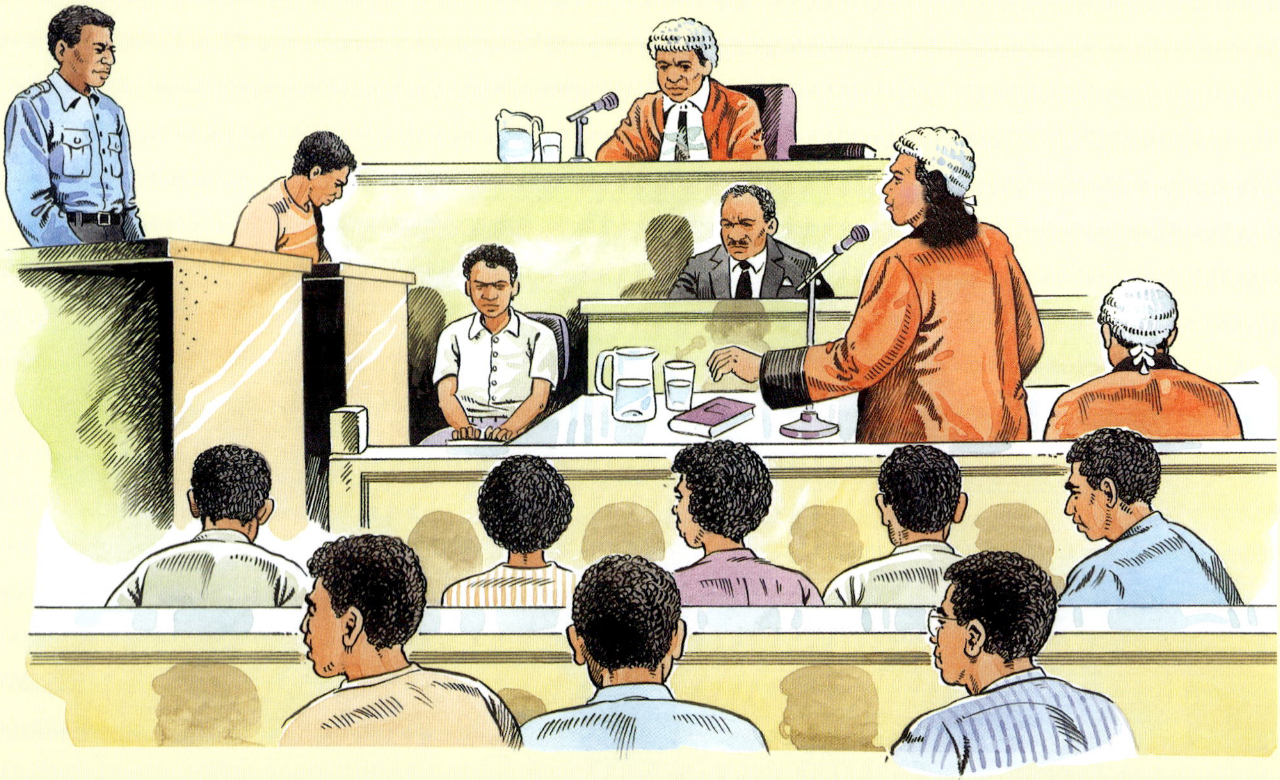

VALUES BEHIND RULES AND LAWS

Rules and laws are based on the values of the community. For example, they should:

- help people to live a healthy way of life
- encourage sharing and helping each other
- be based on Christian values
- help people to live as a community and to work together
- develop a feeling of safety in the community
- help to preserve customs and traditions

Respecting rights and freedoms

The way that we behave affects other people. If we do exactly as we please without thinking about others, then other people will not be happy because our behaviour may be stopping them doing what they want to do. They will think that it is not fair and there will be a lot of trouble in the family or in the community. We sometimes say that people have rights and the freedom to do what they want—as long as this does not take away the rights and freedom of other people to do what *they* want. There has to be a balance between getting what we want and letting other people have what they want.

When we are selfish and think only about ourselves, the following can happen:

- lack of respect for individuals
- breakdown of law and order in the community
- bribery and corruption—people being greedy, dishonest and helping themselves
- fear of violence and fighting in the community
- loss of faith in the courts to do their job properly
- loss of trust in community leaders

When we think about the rights and freedoms of other people before we do what we want to do, there is a feeling of *unity* in the community. Then the following can happen:

- laws are followed and respected
- people live and behave peacefully
- people find solutions to problems
- conflict is resolved or settled
- different points of view are respected

For you to try

- A Choose one of the following: your family, school, village or community. Make a set of rules for the group you have chosen. If there is already a set of rules for the group, then say how you would improve those rules. Can any of the rules be removed from the list?
- What is the purpose of a set of rules or laws?
- Write down some ways in which the community can support and encourage rules and laws.
- Discuss and list the rights of individuals and the standards of behaviour that relate to those rights. The following table may help you—one or two examples have already been included.

The rights of individuals	Standards of behaviour
Money or other things will not be stolen	Being honest, fair, trustworthy, respecting each other

- In a group, discuss the reasons why some people think only about themselves and act against the rights of other people in the community.
- A Write a letter to a friend to explain what happens when the rights and freedom of people are taken away by the action of another person.
- Describe the feeling of unity in your community. What behaviour and what activities would help the feeling of unity to grow?

6 GRADE 8
Relationships

Chapter Summary

In this chapter you will have an opportunity to:

- ✔ Describe the behaviour that is important to you and the groups to which you belong
- ✔ Find out about the rights that people have when they are in relationships
- ✔ Find out about the different ways that we describe people and how this can affect the way they think about themselves
- ✔ Describe your roles and find out how positive role models can affect the way you carry out your own roles
- ✔ Find out about the way that relationships form, develop and end

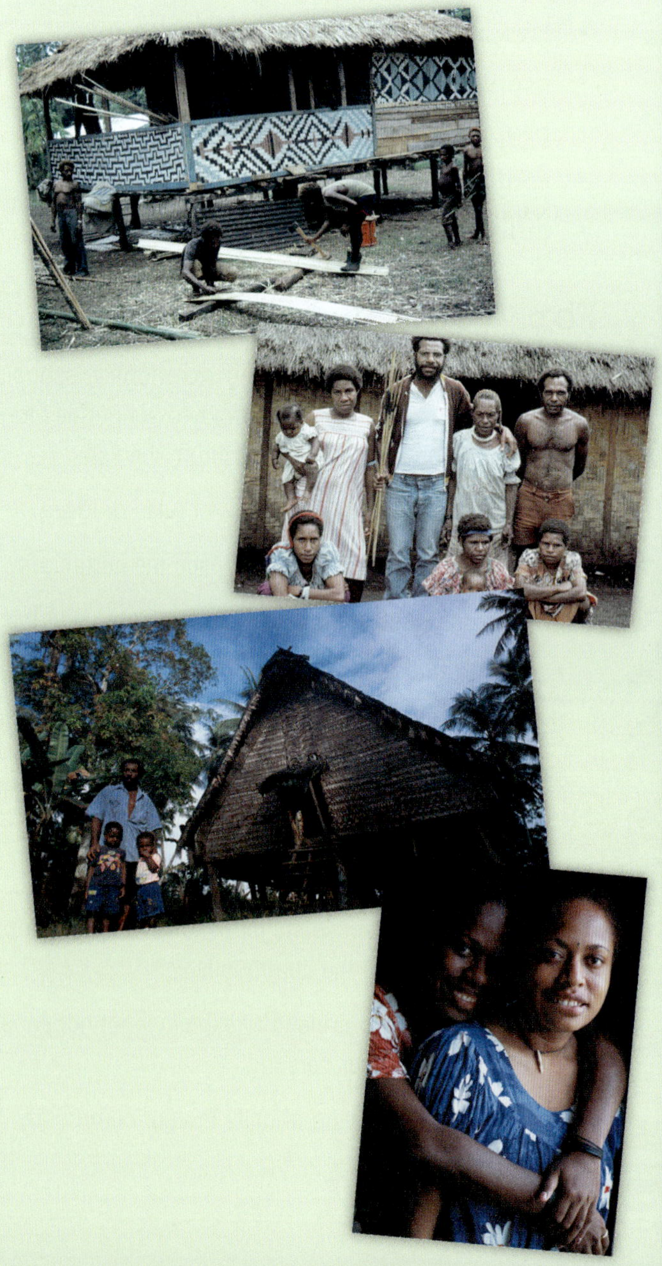

Syllabus references

Strand: Relationships
Sub-strands: Interactions in relationships and groups, cultural and personal identity, changing roles and responsibilities, managing relationships

Outcomes:
- 8.1.1 Describe the standards of behaviour that are important to their community and to families and groups to which they belong
- 8.1.2 Examine the rights of individuals in different forms of relationships
- 8.1.3 Explain how different ways of describing people influence how people value and treat themselves and others
- 8.1.4 Outline their current roles and responsibilities and consider how positive role models can affect how they carry out these roles
- 8.1.5 Describe ways in which relationships form, develop, adapt and end

Interaction in relationships and groups SS

STANDARDS OF BEHAVIOUR

Key facts

- We all belong to a family, to a community and to different groups. Each family, community and group has its own standards of behaviour that are important.
- Behaviour can be assertive, aggressive or submissive.
- The individuals in different relationships have rights. When the rights of people in a relationship are respected, then there can be equality in relationships.
- Ways of describing people can influence how people value and treat themselves and others.
- When we take on a particular role we need certain characteristics, and we can learn these from role models.
- Relationships pass through a number of stages: relationships form, they develop, adapt and end.

We all belong to a family, to a community and to different groups. Each family, community and group has its own standards of behaviour that are important and that members of the group are expected to follow. For example:

- Members of the group are expected to show respect for each other, should be open with each other and should be able to trust each other.
- Each group will have standards about the type and amount of physical contact between members of the group. Some groups will have a lot of physical contact and others will have much less. This is sometimes called the **level of intimacy** between members of the group.
- Members of the group are usually expected to be positive. A person with negative attitudes will not be helpful or popular in the group.
- A member of a group may have to stand up for his or her own rights on occasions.

- Each member of the group should be ready to listen to other members of the group.
- Group members should be able to make good decisions.
- Group members should be able to give and accept compliments.

Members of a group sometimes show the following kinds of behaviour:

Assertive behaviour

Sometimes we might feel that other people do not understand our side of the story or may not be listening carefully enough to what we are saying. We have to speak up for ourselves or stand up for our rights by speaking with confidence. This is called being **assertive**. At the same time, when people make criticisms, we need to learn to deal with these in a positive way. If people criticise us then we should not let it affect our self-esteem or the way we feel about ourselves.

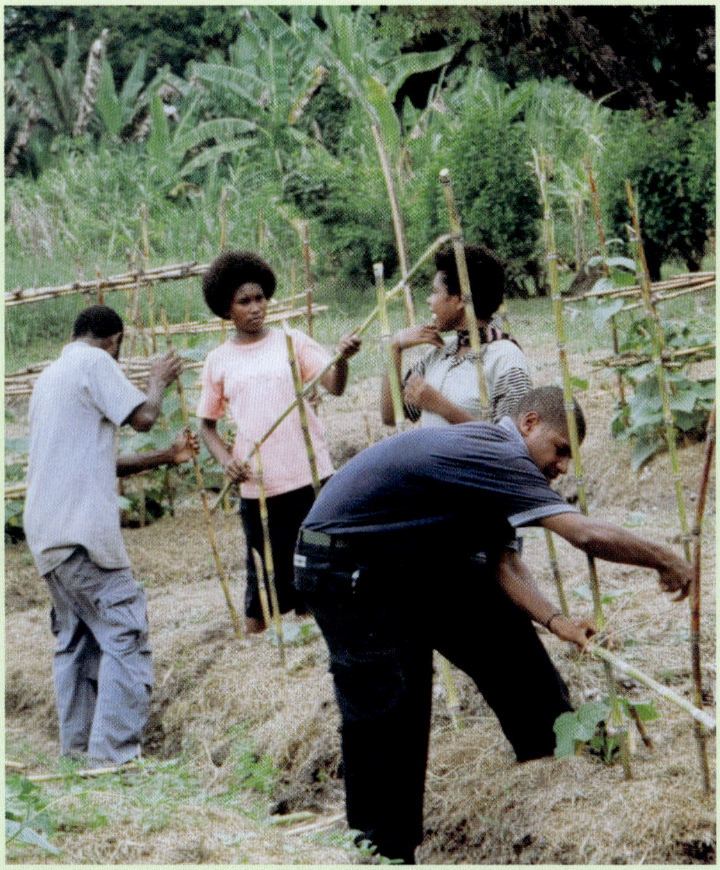

Aggressive behaviour

People may behave in a way that does not consider your feelings or the feelings of others. They may talk very strongly, and other people may feel scared or threatened by this. This is called **aggressive behaviour**. When people are too assertive they can become aggressive. Aggressive behaviour can make some people feel very uncomfortable and can lead to fighting or violence. People who are aggressive sometimes like to have power over other people. They may have high self-esteem but they are not using their self-esteem in a positive way.

Submissive behaviour

Sometimes people can agree very easily even though they don't want to, or they may be very slow at making decisions, or they may pretend that concerns or issues are not important when they are. These are all examples of **submissive behaviour**. People who are submissive are not always treated equally or fairly in a relationship and may not get what they want.

If we are submissive then we are too passive and may not feel good about ourselves—being submissive is not good for our self-esteem. Sometimes we know that we should not be so submissive but we still do not give our opinion or tell others what we would like. We all need to be appropriately assertive. This means that we need to learn how to be more active and try to make things happen rather than just allowing things to happen.

We can show these three types of behaviour on a scale as follows:

SUBMISSIVE (Passive)	ASSERTIVE	AGGRESSIVE (Active)

For you to try

- Prepare a two-minute talk to give to the class about the reasons why we have rules in the family.
- In small groups, discuss the reasons or the behaviour that make a relationship a good one or a bad one. Write down the main ideas that you discuss.
- Write down some different cultural and personal values. How do these values influence relationships?

RIGHTS OF INDIVIDUALS IN DIFFERENT RELATIONSHIPS

All communities have rules and laws that are based on the values of the community—the things that people say or believe are important. The beliefs in what is right and fair and the laws of the community give people certain **rights**. Without these beliefs and laws we would not have the rights that allow us to enjoy life and to be free and happy.

People in different countries have different rights that depend on the conditions in each country. When we have rights we do not always think about them or even know that we have that right, but when the right is taken away, then we will feel the loss of that right. In Papua New Guinea people have the following rights. Because rights of individuals are so important, they are included in the constitution of Papua New Guinea.

Your Rights

The right to have a name and a nationality—to belong to Papua New Guinea as a country

The right to think for yourself

The right to speak freely for yourself

The right to be free from discrimination—so that people will not judge you because of the place you are from, or your beliefs, or the church that you belong to

The right to life—so that no one should take away your life

The right to be healthy and to have health services

The right to a fair standard of living

The right to parents who take good care of their children

The right to have an education

The right to protection from being treated badly

The right to choose good leaders and to change those leaders

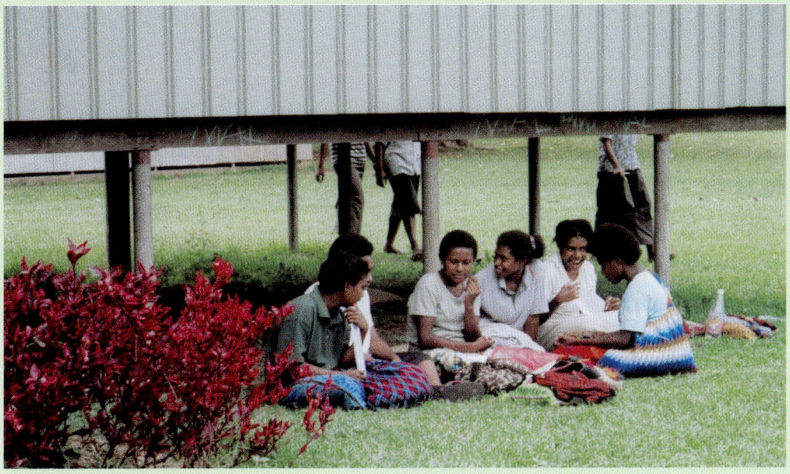

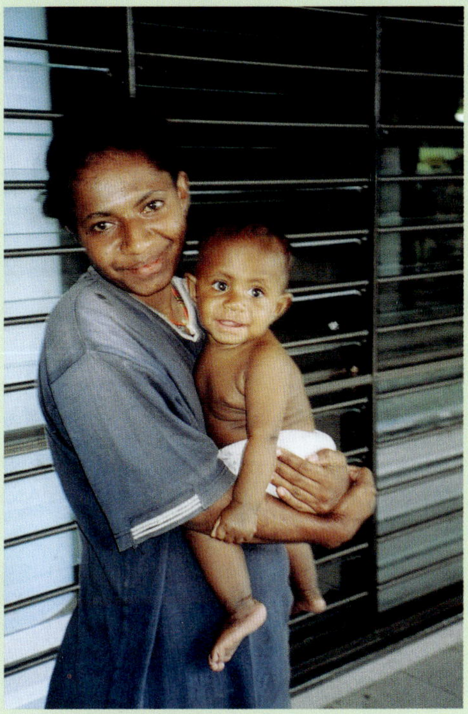

Rights of a citizen of PNG

The four basic rights are:

Freedom to make your own decisions and to go where you want

To live safely and securely in healthy conditions

Protection by the law

Freedom from cruel and violent treatment

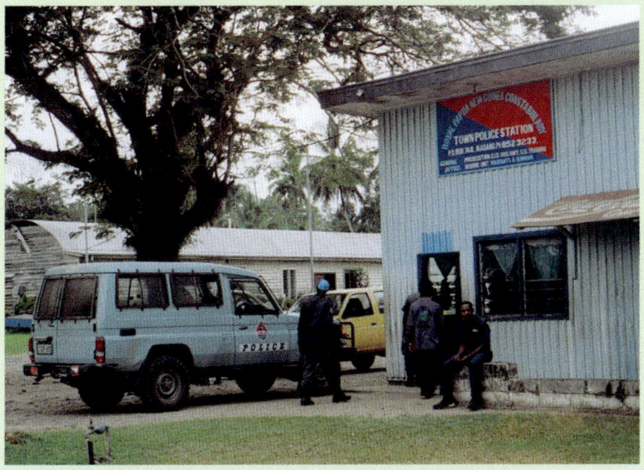

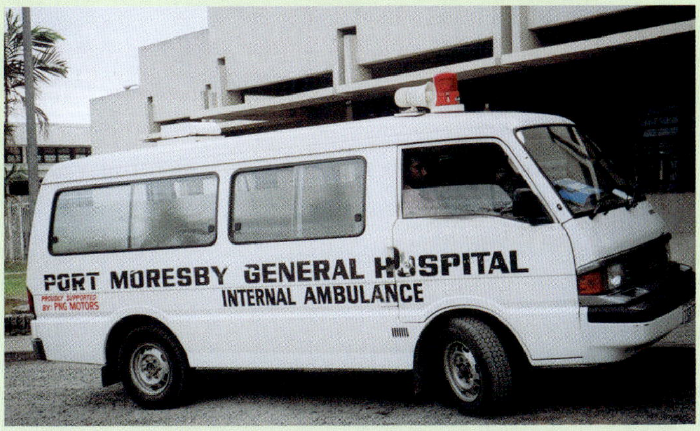

EQUALITY IN RELATIONSHIPS

We all have relationships with different people. Our first relationships are with our families at home, and when we go to school we begin to make relationships with other students and with the teachers. Relationships will begin to develop with people that we meet and continue to meet regularly. However, both people in a relationship must be interested in continuing to be part of the relationship. For example, for two people to be friends, both people must be interested in being friends. If someone does not want to be friends with you, then it is hard to have a friendship with that person.

In relationships between friends, and in other types of relationship, there should be **equality**. This means that both people in a relationship should be equally important and have the same amount of power. One person should not be always telling the other person what to do or making all the decisions about what they will do. When men and women go to work, there should be equality between men and women in the place where they work. For example, if men and women do the same work, they should be paid the same amount of money.

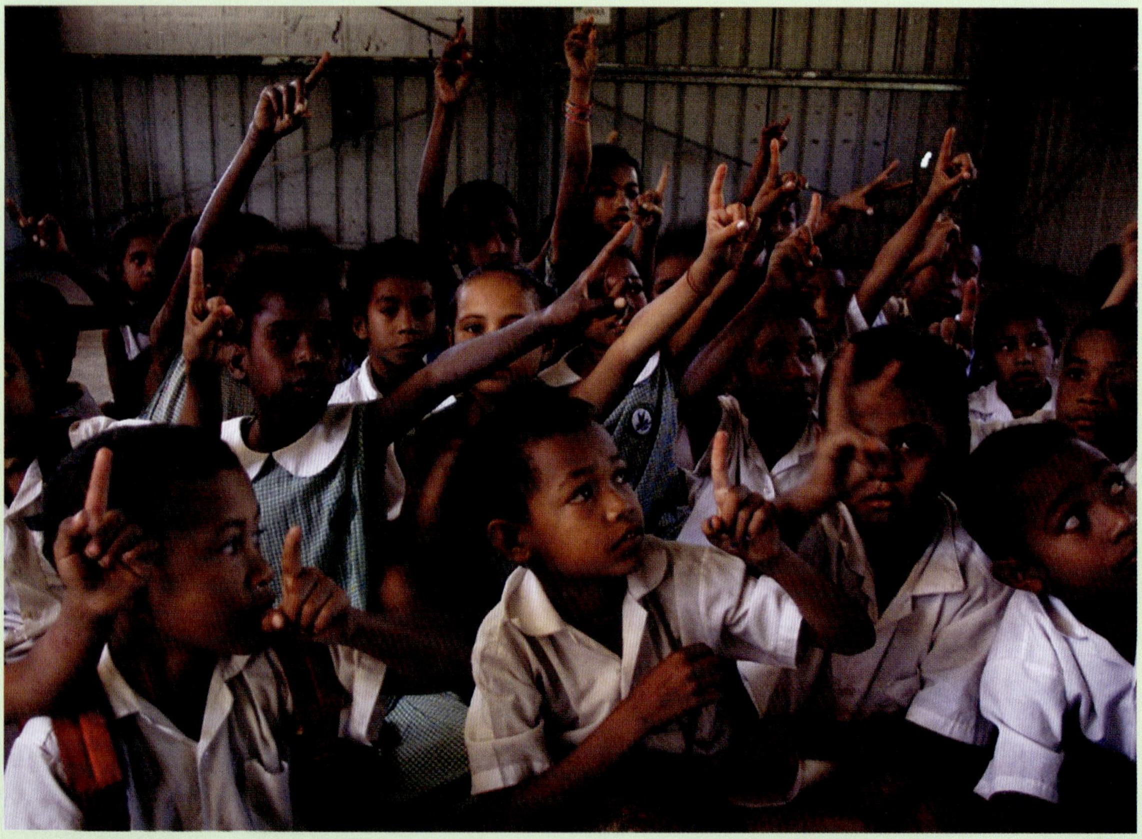

When one person tries to be more important than the other, or tells the other person what to do, or makes the other person look small, then we say that there is **inequality** in the relationship. Other examples of inequality are when one person is very aggressive and the other is very quiet and passive, or when one person is very dependent on another person. When there is inequality in a relationship then one person may not be happy about that relationship, and this can lead to conflict.

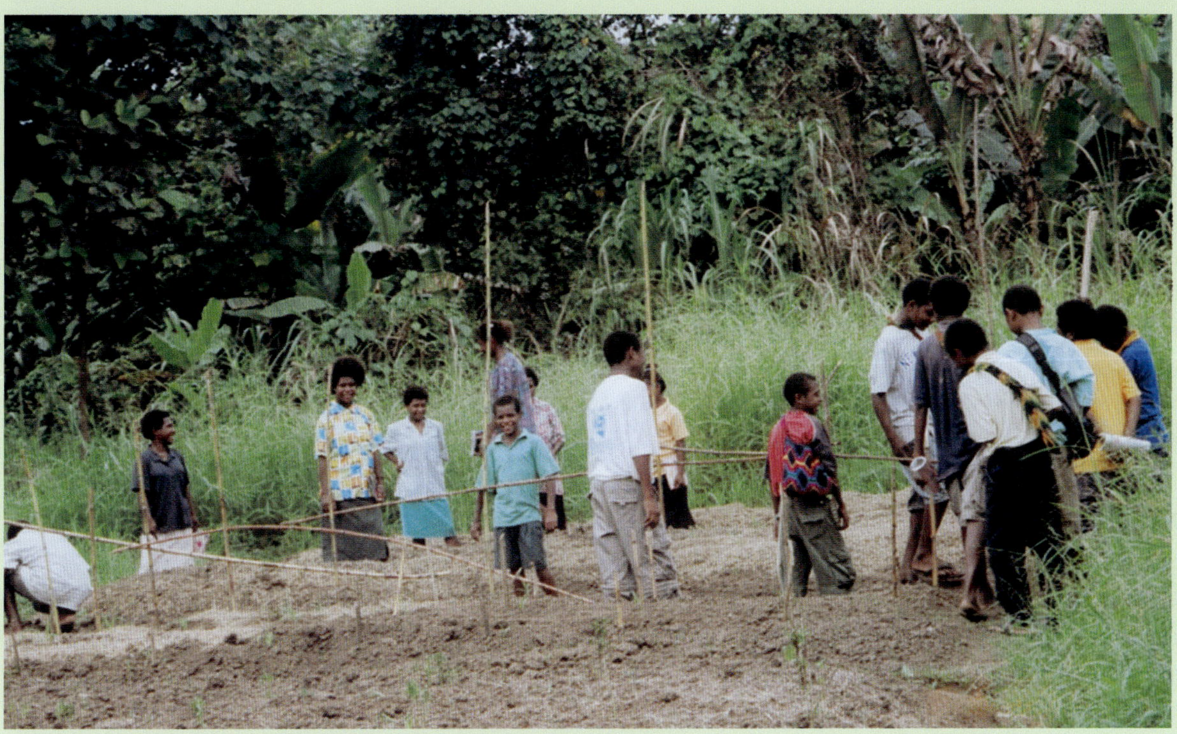

Equality in relationships is important at school, at home and at work

For you to try

- Make groups of boys and girls and discuss the following: How can we make sure that boys and girls, men and women, are treated equally? Each group reports back to the whole class.
- Think about a relationship that you know well. Give examples to show the equality or inequality in the relationship. Use the following table:

Examples of equality	Examples of inequality

- Find out about laws that give equal rights to men and women. What can we do to make sure that the law is followed?
- What rights do people have? How do the rights of individuals affect relationships?

Cultural and personal identity

WAYS OF DESCRIBING PEOPLE

We all need to be able to describe each other, and the way that we do this can be funny or serious, kind or unkind. For example, if we are describing the physical appearance of a person, or the way they look, we might say that they are tall or short, fat or thin, big or small. If the person is very tall, we might make fun about their head being in the clouds.

We might describe the way that they behave towards other people. We might say that a person is friendly, honest and caring, or angry, aggressive and bossy.

When we describe other people, we often talk about how smart they are and whether they are quick, slow, clever or practical. When teachers and adults talk about children, they sometimes use these words because they show how well young people can learn to do different things.

We sometimes use parts of the person's culture to describe them, such as their clothes or the decorations that they are wearing.

We need to be careful when we describe people because the words that we use can be positive or negative. Even if we believe something is true, we can still hurt someone if we say exactly what we think without considering his or her feelings. For example, if we say something about the shape of the body of another person we can hurt the person.

We also need to be careful that we do not give an opinion or make a judgment about somebody without having good reasons. This is called **stereotyping**. For example, if you have been told that all people from a particular place have a certain appearance or behave in particular way, then you may

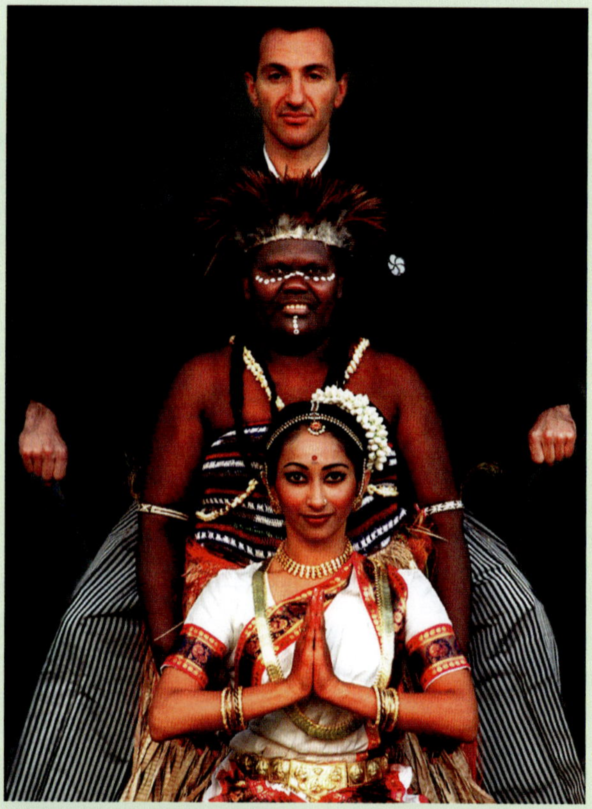

Dancers from different cultures

form an opinion about that person without trying to find out for yourself what they are like. All people from one group are not the same, and if you keep an open mind you will then be able to decide for yourself rather than making up your mind without good reasons.

When we make up our minds without good reason and treat a person unfairly, then we are discriminating against that person. **Discrimination** is unfair and is against the law in many countries, including Papua New Guinea. For example, in some countries it is against the law to discriminate against people because of the colour of their skin.

Stereotyping and discrimination are important because they can affect our choices and decisions, even though there is no good reason to make those choices or decisions. For example, stereotyping and discrimination can affect the following:

- the food that you eat
- the way that you dress
- the type of friends that you choose
- the place where you live
- the sport that you play
- the work that you choose to do
- the person that you marry

RESPECTING OTHER PEOPLE

When we meet other people it is important to respect the ways that people are different. People from different cultures have different ideas about the way that things should be done, and in Papua New Guinea there are many unique cultures. We want other people to respect our culture and in return we need to respect the culture of others. When people respect the different ways of doing things that we have, then we say there is **tolerance** and people are more likely to live happily together.

For you to try

- Choose someone that you know and write a description of that person. In what ways is the person typical of the groups to which he or she belongs and in what ways is he or she unusual?
- In small groups, discuss how you feel when other people use stereotyping and discrimination against you.
- Think about some examples of stereotyping or discrimination that you have seen or heard about. Copy and complete the following table:

Example of stereotyping or discrimination (Who was involved? What happened?)	**What was the effect on the person?**

- Write a story to describe how stereotypes and discrimination can affect a person's sense of identity and relationships.

Changing roles and responsibilities

POSITIVE ROLE MODELS

In most communities there are people who are admired and respected because of the things that they have done in the past and the things that they continue to do. For example, we might admire people who are very good at sport or people who play music, or we might admire people who have been successful in their education or in their job.

These people that we look up to are called **role models** because we often want to be like them. Role models might be well known in your province, in Papua New Guinea or in the world. However, a role model might also just be someone who is not well known but whom you admire. For example, you might admire and respect an auntie who has never been to school but who works very hard for her family and is always cheerful and makes fun even when life is difficult.

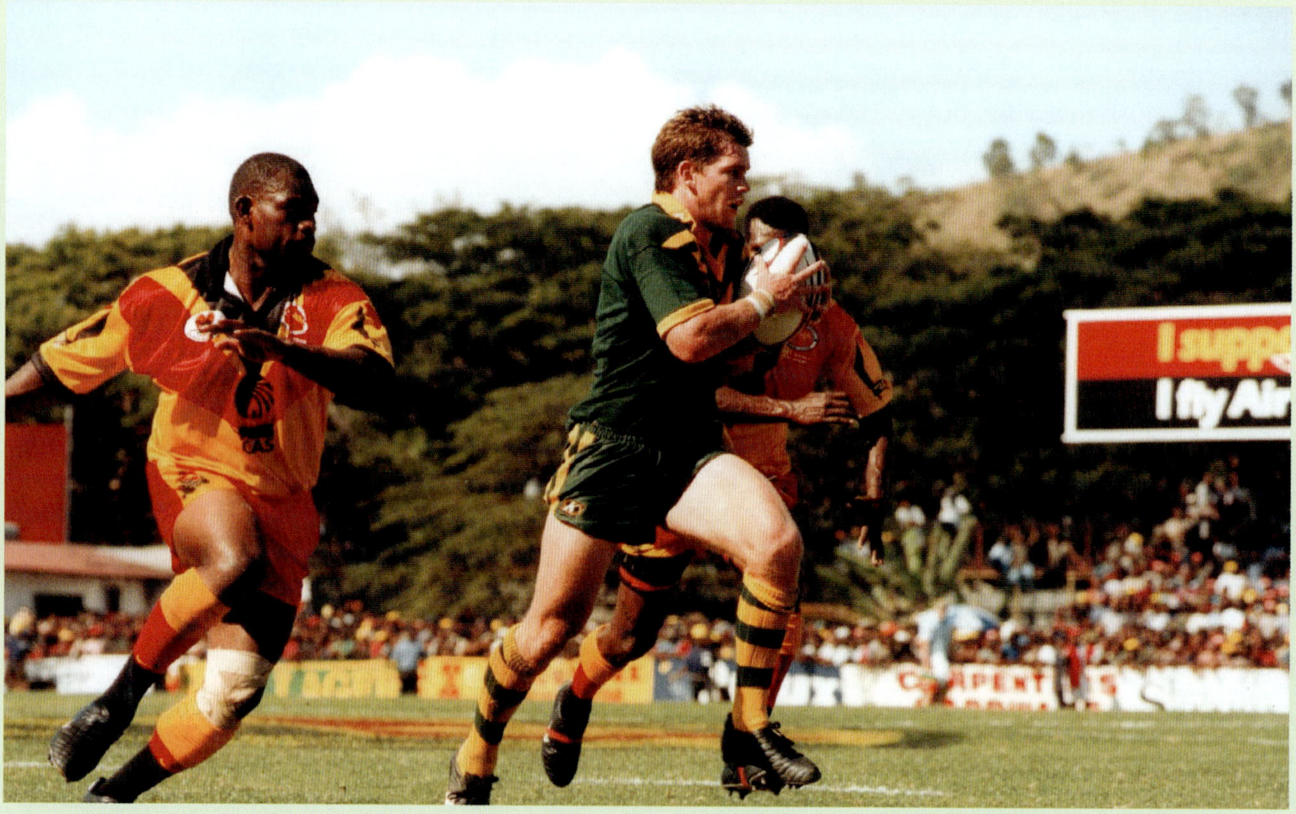

Some characteristics of role models are:

- having a dream or a goal
- facing up to problems
- being well organised
- recovering from setbacks when things go wrong
- having persistence and determination to keep going and not to give up easily

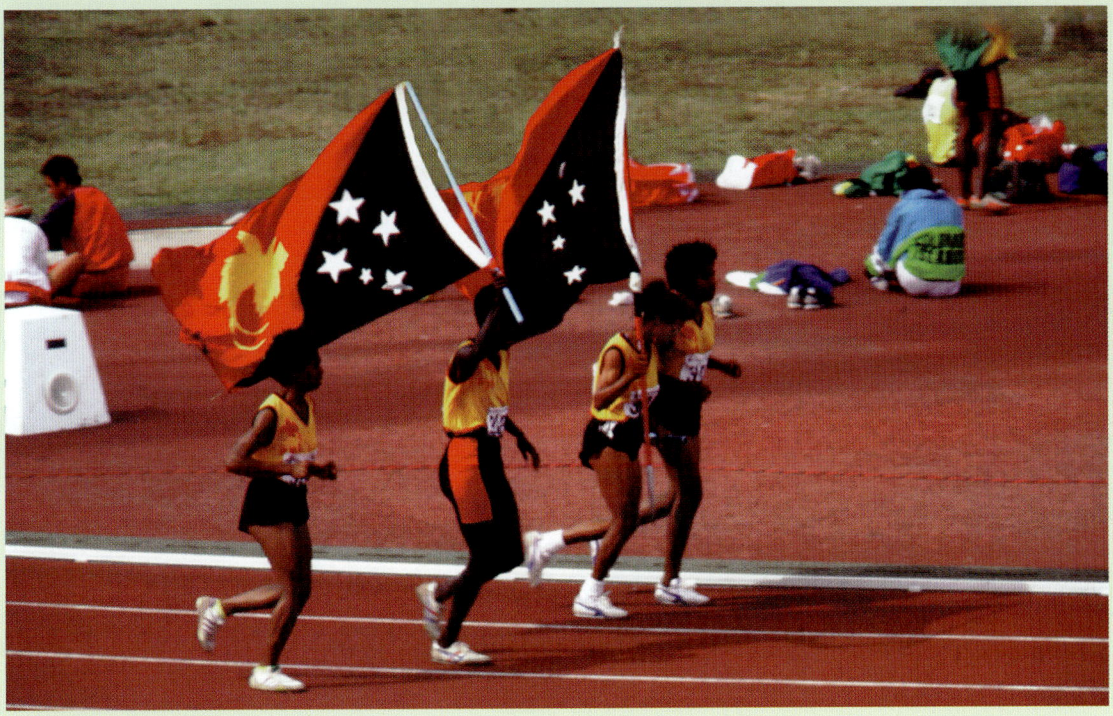

YOUR CURRENT ROLE

We all have different roles at different times in our lives that may need different characteristics. In your current role as a student and a young person in your community, the following characteristics will help you:

- confidence
- courtesy
- determination
- trying hard to do well or to achieve excellence
- flexibility
- being organised
- facing up to problems
- having a dream or a goal

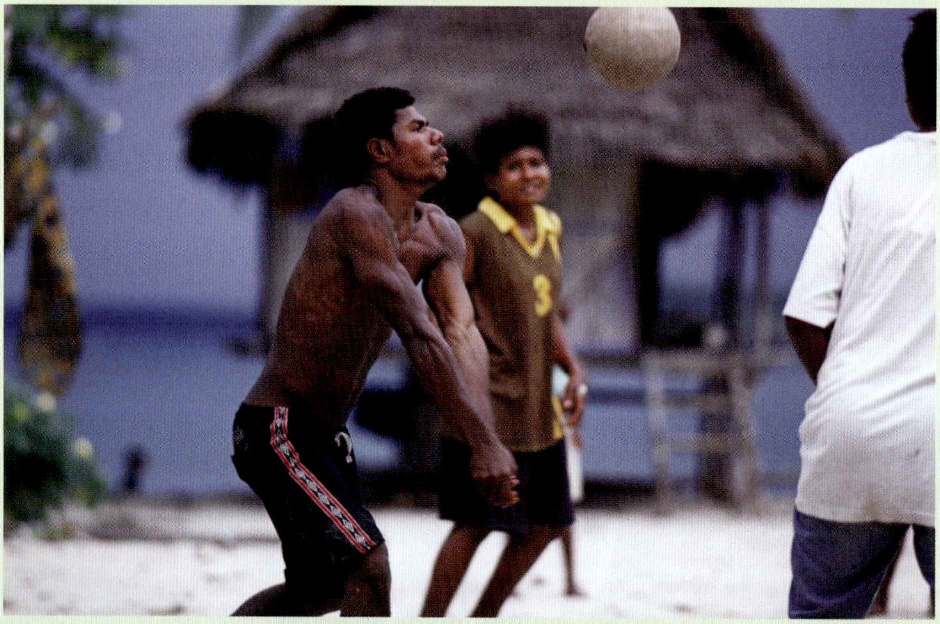

For you to try

- Find out from your friends who their male and female role models are, and get them to give reasons for choosing them. Boys may not be interested in female role models and girls may not be interested in male role models, but you still need to find out about both by talking to each other. You could use a table like the one below:

Male role models	Reasons for choosing this role model

Female role models	Reasons for choosing this role model

Compare the male and female role models. What are the reasons for the differences?

- List and discuss some of the characteristics of positive role models.
- Choose a role model that you want to follow. Give reasons for your choice and write down some characteristics that your role model does not have.

Managing relationships

HOW RELATIONSHIPS START, DEVELOP AND END (ML)

Relationships are important to all of us and at times can be great fun or make you very sad and upset. The first relationships we have are with our family members and, of course, we cannot choose who they will be. However, as we get older we begin to choose our own friends. We begin to choose those people with whom we want to develop a relationship. Most of us will choose to make friends with someone who is about the same age as us and who has interests that are similar to ours. In other words, we usually begin to form relationships when we have some things in common, although occasionally two people who are very different from each other may start to make friends and get on very well together.

After a relationship has started, it will continue to develop if the two people treat each other in certain ways. For example, in a good relationship people show each other the following:

- respect
- courtesy
- compassion
- kindness
- patience
- love
- generosity
- loyalty
- trust
- forgiveness.

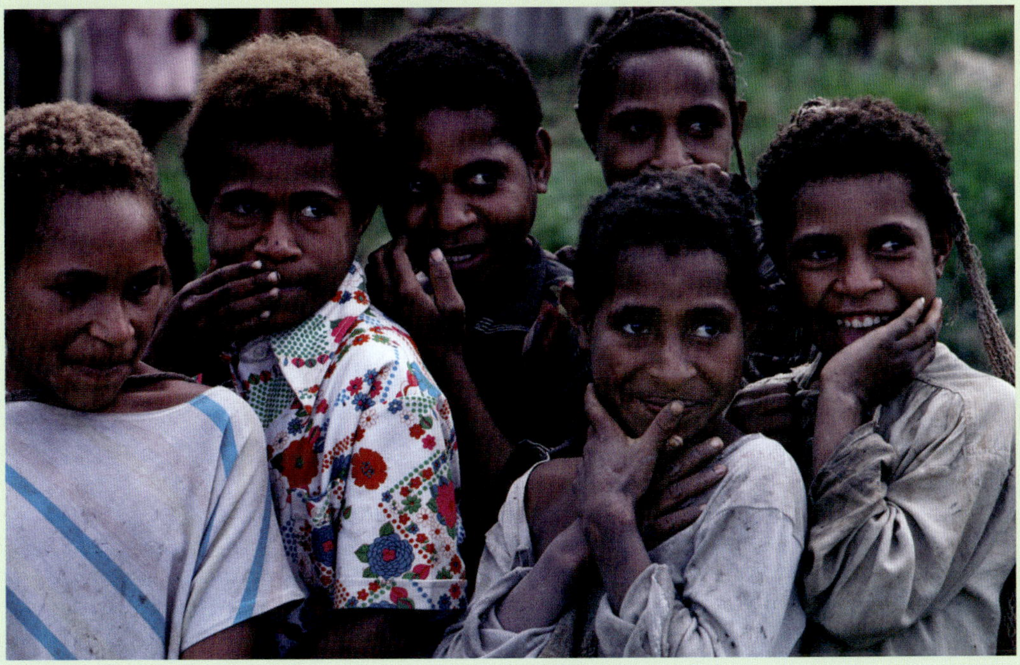

Relationships and friendships can change when someone moves away, or when they learn new skills or complete or achieve something. For example, if two friends both want to join the same sports team or both want to pass the same exam, and one is successful and one is unsuccessful, then the relationship between the two friends may change. The successful person might feel pleased for himself or herself but sad for the friend, and the unsuccessful person might feel pleased for his or her friend but also jealous of that friend's success.

We can adjust to these sorts of changes in a number of ways. For example, if someone moves away we can continue to communicate with him or her and maybe even visit from time to time. When our friends are having problems we can listen to each other, accept support from each other, share our ideas and continue to celebrate when we have a success or a birthday.

Some relationships and friendships last for many years but others may last for a much shorter time. Sometimes people who are in a relationship just slowly drift apart so that they do less things together and do not feel so close to one another. When a relationship changes gradually people may have time to get used to the change, although they still may not like it. Sometimes one person may do something that hurts the other person or one person may just decide to suddenly end the relationship. It can be a very hard time when a relationship ends, and people who are feeling hurt need our understanding and support.

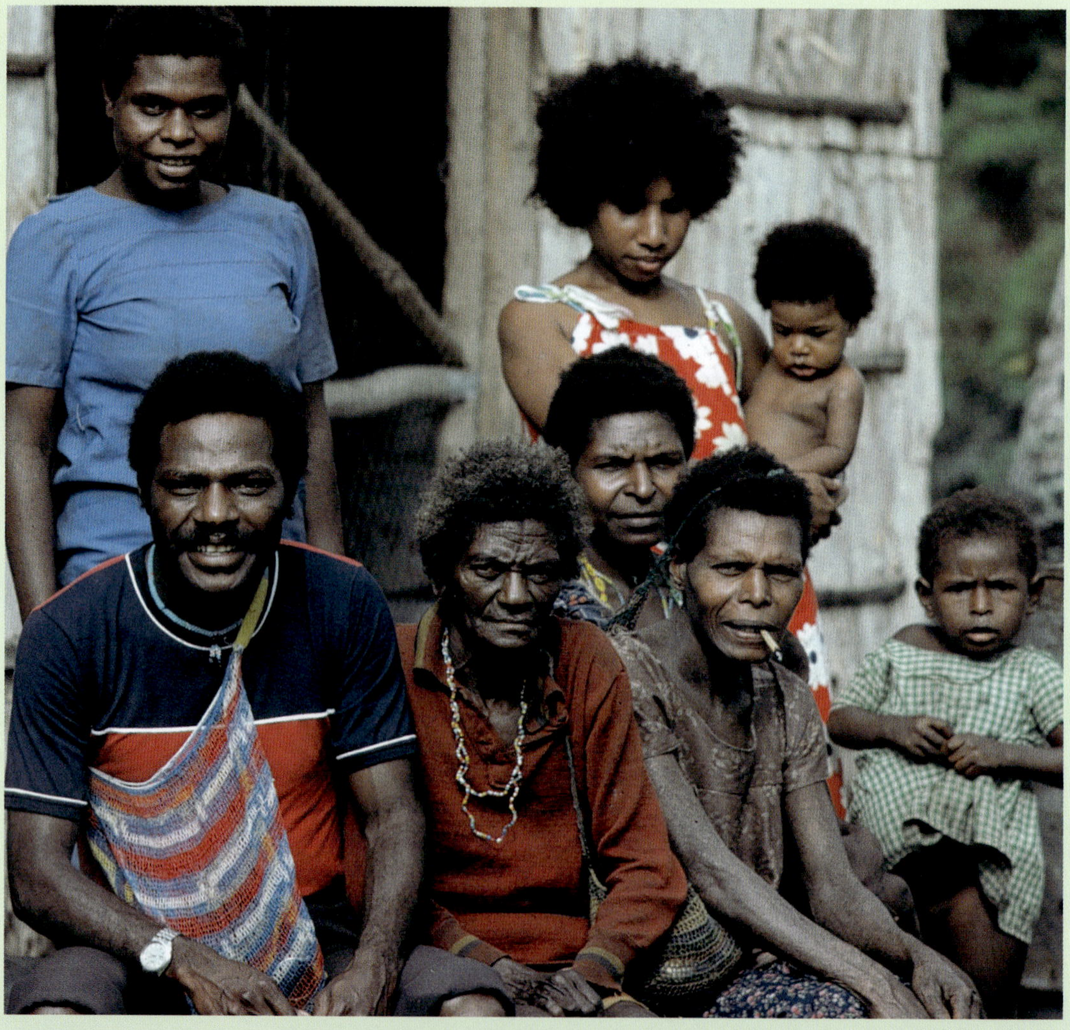

For you to try

- What do you think makes a good friendship? Make a list of the characteristics of a good friendship.
- Discuss how new relationships are formed and how to adjust to the changes and needs of a relationship.
- If you have to end a relationship, how do you do it without hurting the other person?
- Describe some ways to deal with the end of a relationship and the type of support to give to those in need.

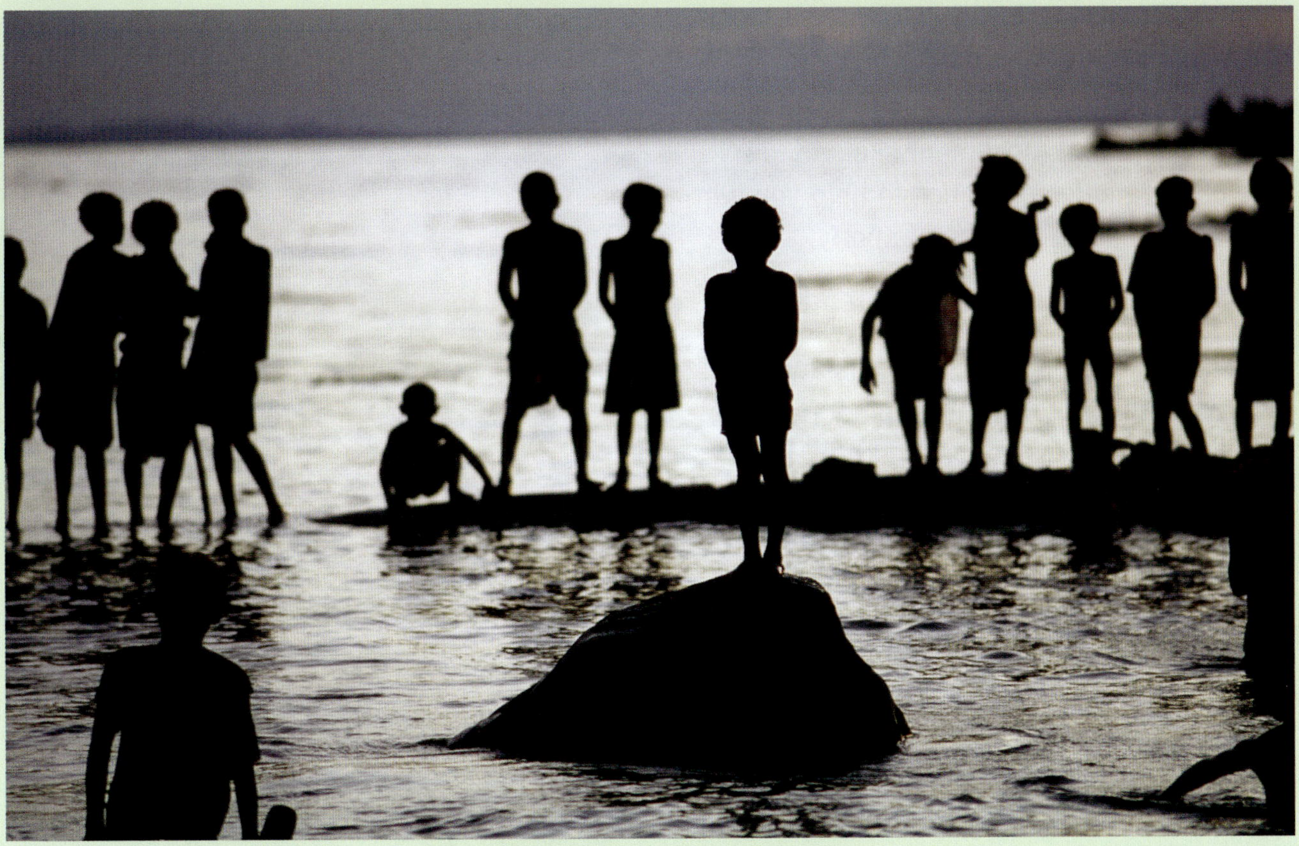

7

Movement and Physical Activity

Chapter Summary

In this chapter you will have an opportunity to:

- ✔ Use different movement skills to carry out strategies or tactics to help you win when playing a game of sport
- ✔ Design a personal fitness program
- ✔ Find out about your strengths and weaknesses when playing sport, and those of other players, and how to improve
- ✔ Learn how to assess risk and follow rules and safety procedures when you play so as to prevent injury
- ✔ Find out more about ways to help people take part in recreation, sporting and leisure activities
- ✔ Learn good ways to communicate and cooperate when you play team games

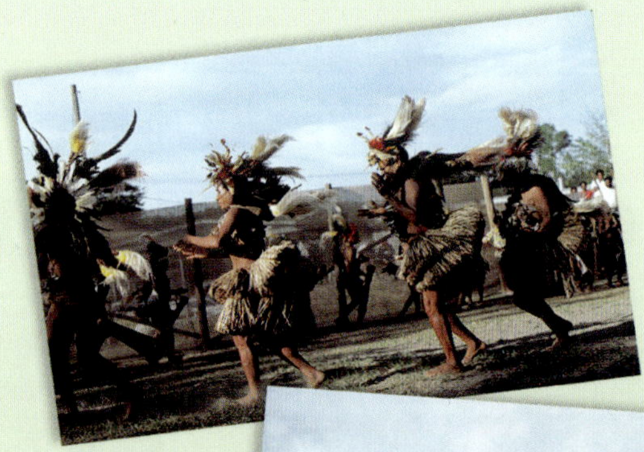

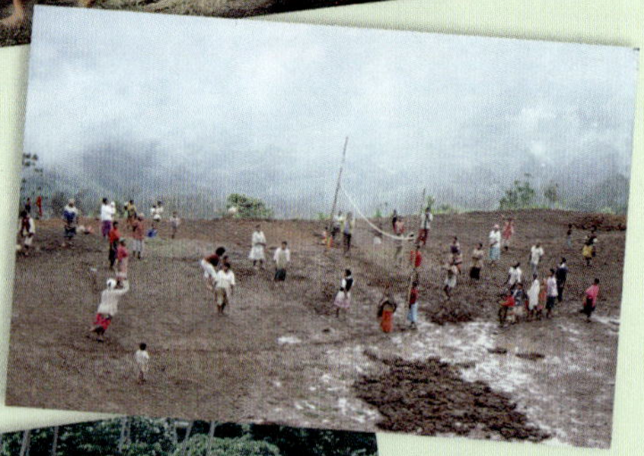

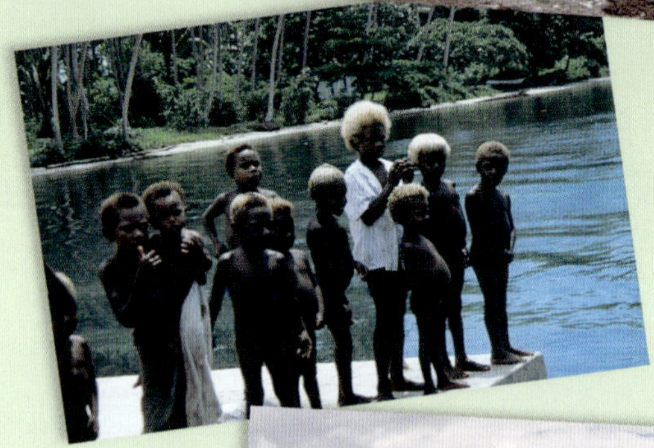

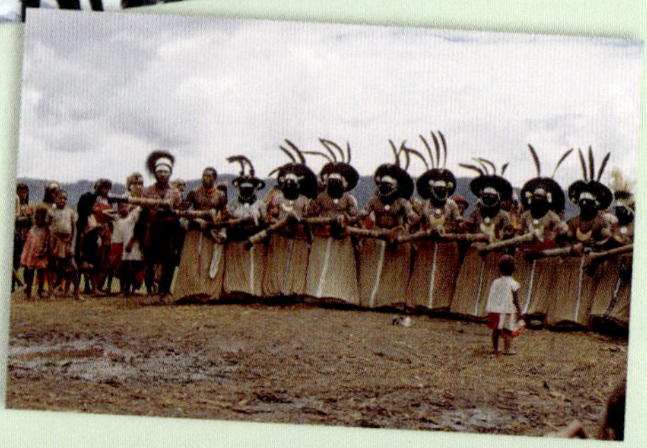

Syllabus references

Strand: Movement and physical activity
Sub-strands: Movement skills, fitness for health, safety, leisure and recreation, roles and responsibilities

Outcomes:

8.2.1 Implement strategies in games adapting a range of locomotor skills

8.2.2 Provide feedback on the performance of oneself and others based on movement control, and improve performance in a game

8.2.3 Design a personal fitness program

8.2.4 Demonstrate behaviour that influences personal safety of others in games and play

8.2.5 Describe how people and facilities influence the choice of recreation, sporting and leisure activities

8.2.6 Develop effective ways of communicating and cooperating in team games

Movement skills

USING STRATEGIES AND TACTICS WHEN PLAYING GAMES

Key facts

- When we take part in games, sports and dance, we need to link a range of different skills together. In order to win we need to link these skills in special ways to make strategies or tactics like attacking and defending.
- All players have strengths and weaknesses. We need to know our own strengths and weaknesses and those of other players. We also need to know how to maintain our strengths and to improve our weaknesses.
- A fitness program is made up of different parts and so can be designed for different individuals.
- Some sporting activities can be dangerous and we need to know how to assess risk and follow rules and safety procedures when we play so as to prevent injury.
- In order to encourage people to take part in recreational and leisure activities, suitable people are needed to organise the activities and suitable facilities are needed.
- When we play games and sport, we need to use suitable ways of communicating and cooperating.

When we play a game or a sport we usually need to combine a number of different skills in a sequence of movements. Beginning to learn a new game or sport can be very frustrating because at first we are not very good and so we do not enjoy what we are doing. If we practise regularly we get better at the activity and our skills develop, so we enjoy it more.

When we take part in a competition and we want to win, we need to put the skills together in a way that makes a **strategy** and uses **tactics**. This means that we have a plan and a way to carry out the plan in order to win.

For example, in sports like soccer, rugby, netball and basketball the players have to get the ball into the other half of the field and score goals, points or tries. The strategy to do this is to attack. Other members of the team may be trying to prevent the other side from scoring goals or tries. The strategy to do this is to defend. Some team members may have to both attack and defend depending on which side has possession of the ball. Everybody has the responsibility to work together as a team and to try to win. The team that has good individual players who work together to carry out the plan or strategy is the one that is most likely to be successful.

When a team is defending, then they need to prevent the other side from scoring. They might do this by making sure there is not enough space to play the ball, or by not giving them enough time and by marking each other.

When a team has a strategy, they sometimes arrange a special signal with the other members of the team so that they know what to do, but the other side does not know. For example, in basketball you might call out a number or word that means that ball is going to be passed from one player to another player and then back to the first player again in order to move the ball around a player from the other team.

A strategy that is well planned and successful is very pleasing for the players to carry out and very enjoyable for spectators to watch. For example, when the ball passes smoothly along a line of rugby players who manage to avoid being tackled and then a try is scored, this is an exciting moment.

Strategies and tactics need to be carefully planned and the players need to practise so that they can coordinate the different skills that are needed. A good coach can help players to develop and practise successful strategies and tactics.

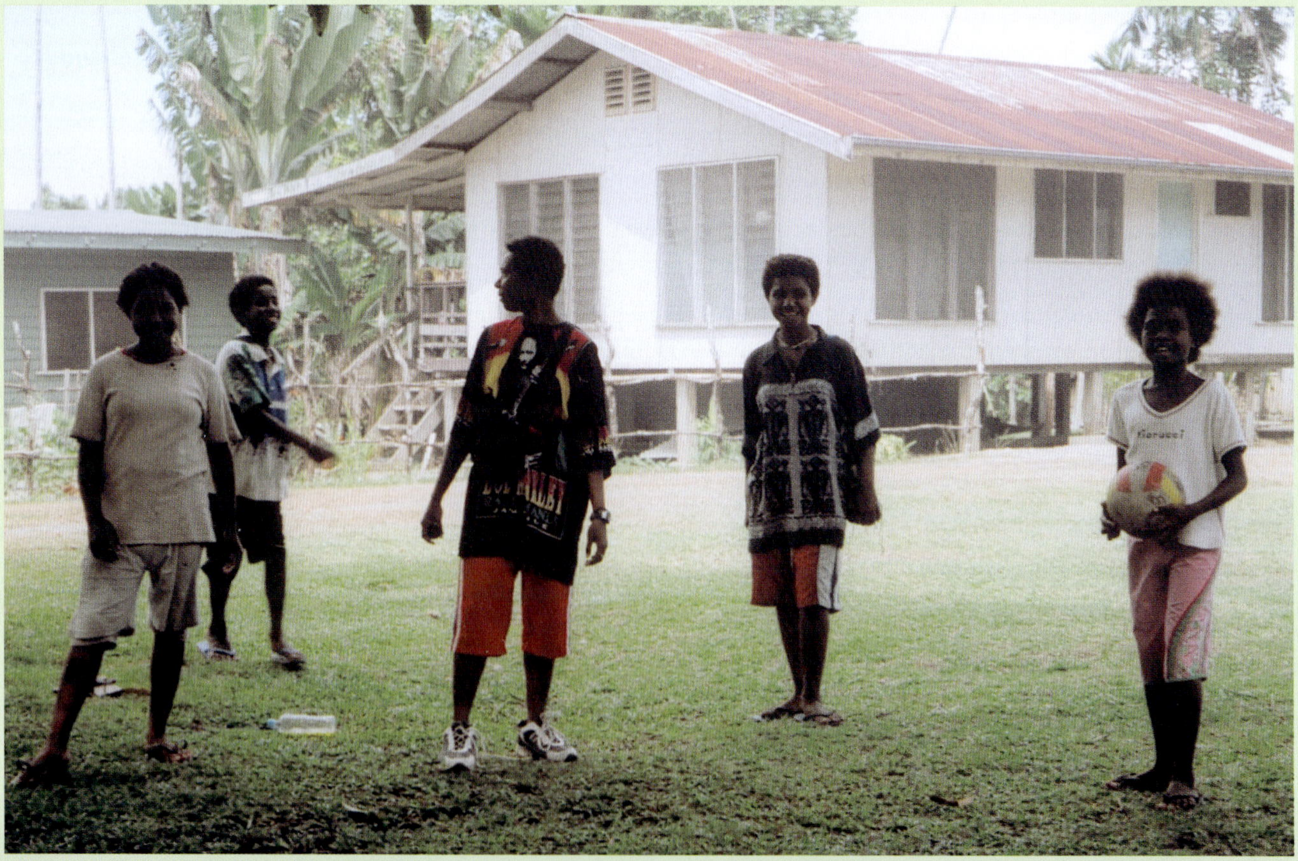

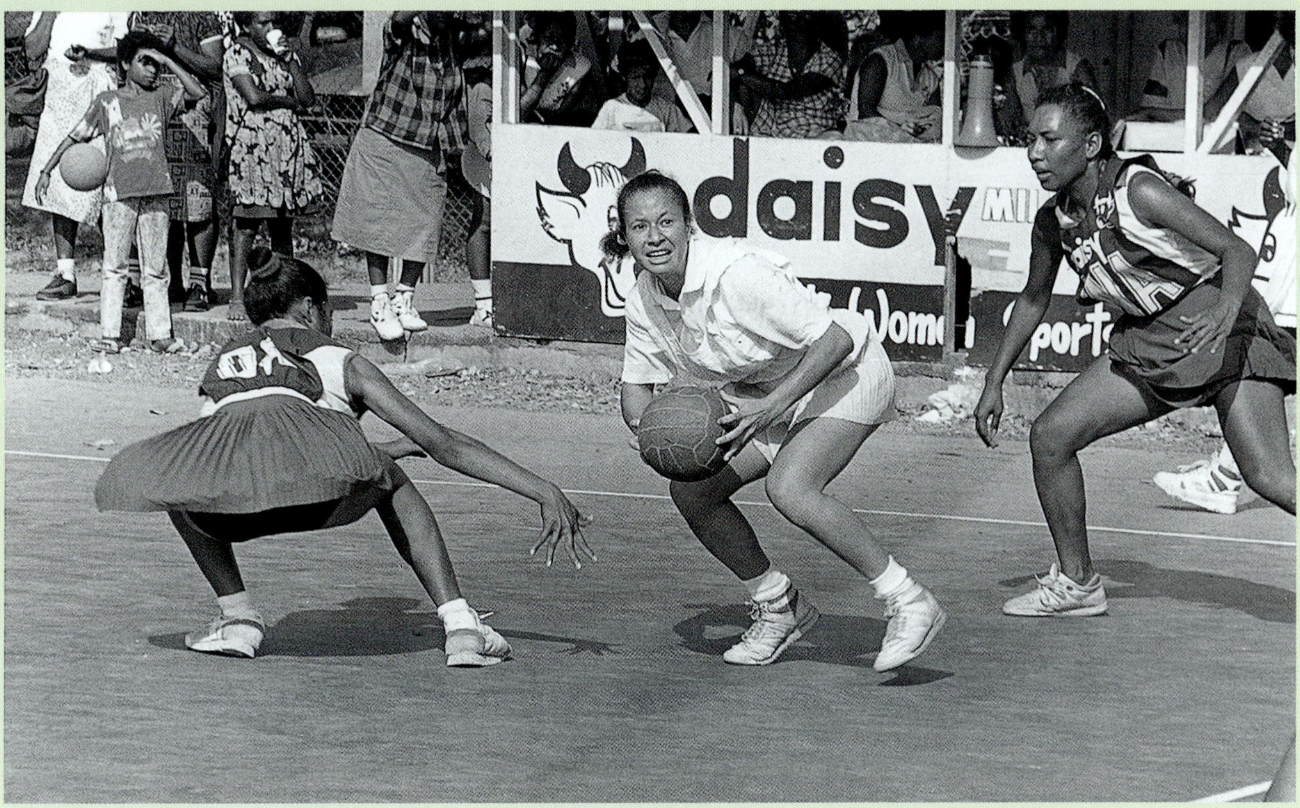

For you to try

- Choose a game that is commonly played in your area. Practise the skills that are needed to develop strategies and tactics for that game.
- Write down the skills that are needed to play a game in the order in which they need to be learned. Explain why you chose the order that you chose.
- Play a game that requires a variety of tactics and skills.
- Evaluate your performance at playing a game and suggest ways to improve on your weaknesses.

COMBINING SKILLS

In all sports people have to be competent at particular skills in order to play the game successfully. For example, when we travel or move from one place to another place then we need to use **locomotor skills**. We usually combine or link together several different skills. For example, we might combine running, jumping, hopping and skipping, or we might need to take off and land using one foot or two feet.

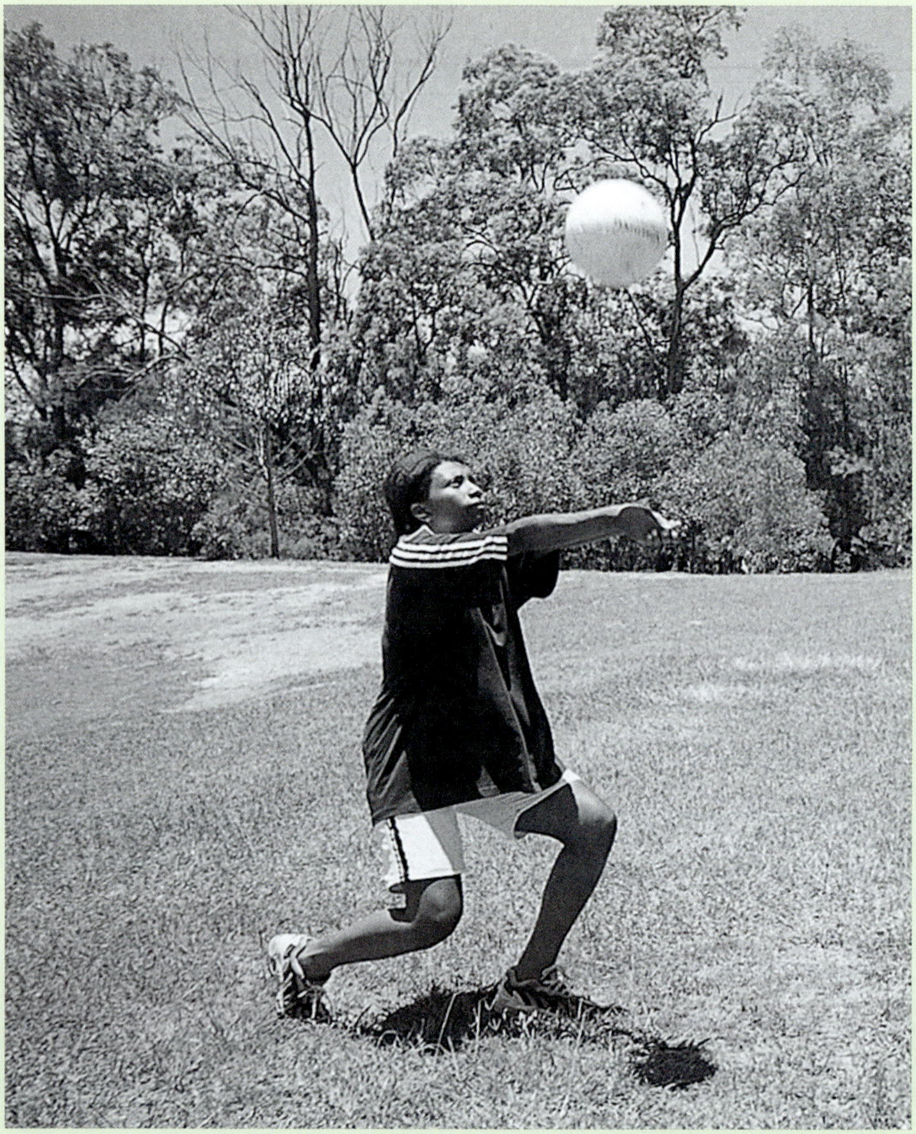

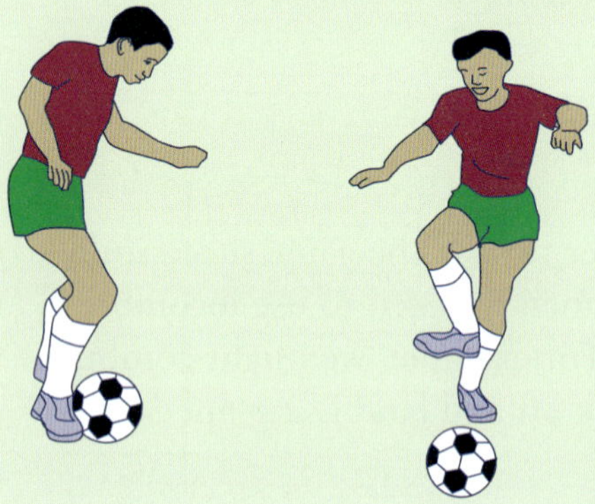

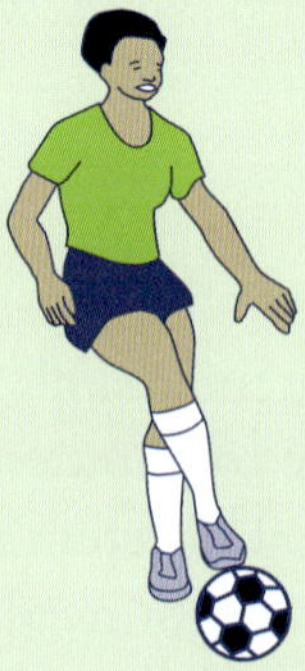

The step-over-the-ball dribble

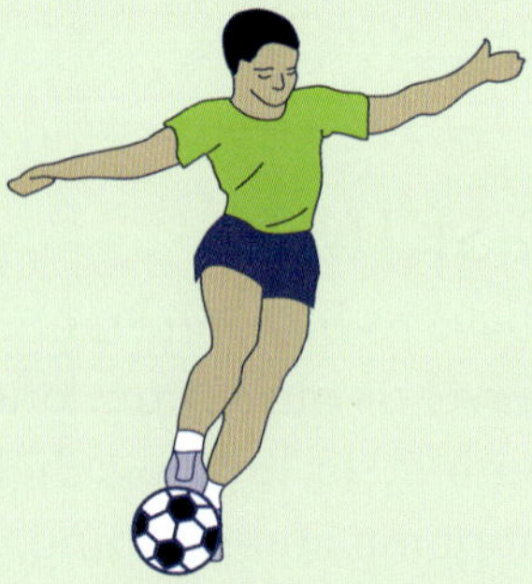

The step-on-the-ball dribble

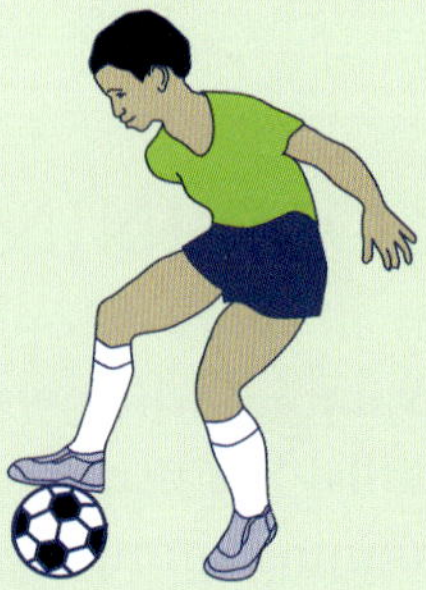

The pull-the-ball-back dribble

Kicking using the inside of the foot

In many sports we need to combine the skills that allow us to move from place to place with other skills such as hitting or catching a ball. For example, when playing netball or basketball we need to move quickly around the court, but we also need to pass the ball and shoot for the goal. However, in basketball we can travel with the ball while in netball we cannot run with the ball and must pass it within three seconds.

The range of skills that are needed in games and sport require body control and coordination. When we become competent in a number of different movement skills it means that we can then take part in a bigger variety of games and sports and get more enjoyment from taking part.

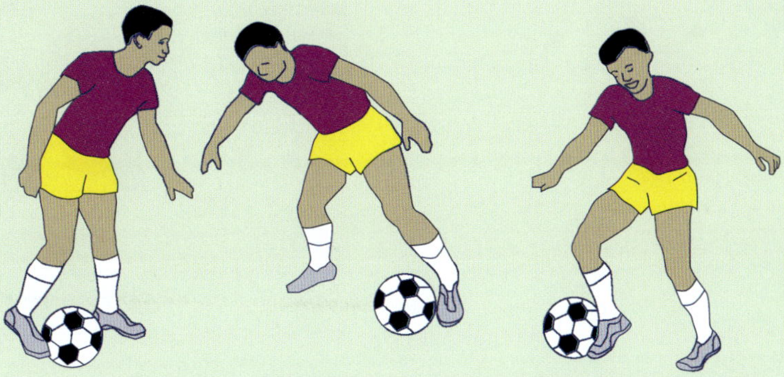

Using the inside of the foot

Using the outside of the foot

Set shot

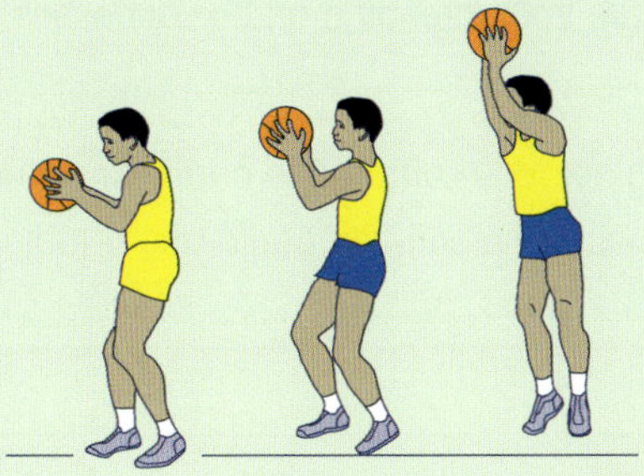

Lay-up shot

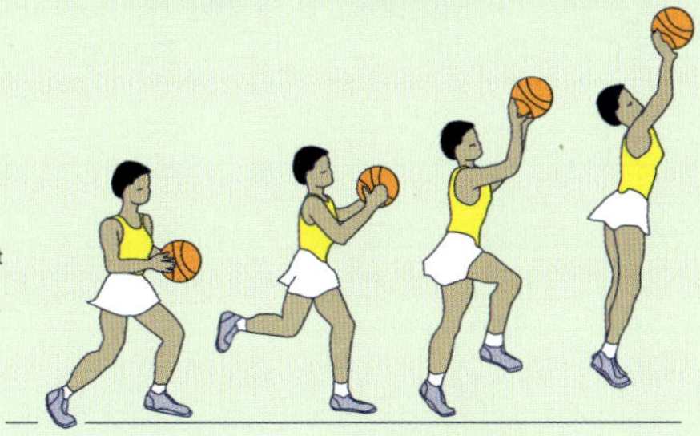

Hook shot

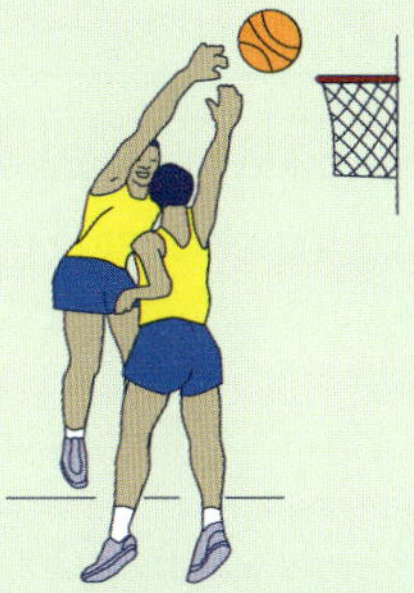

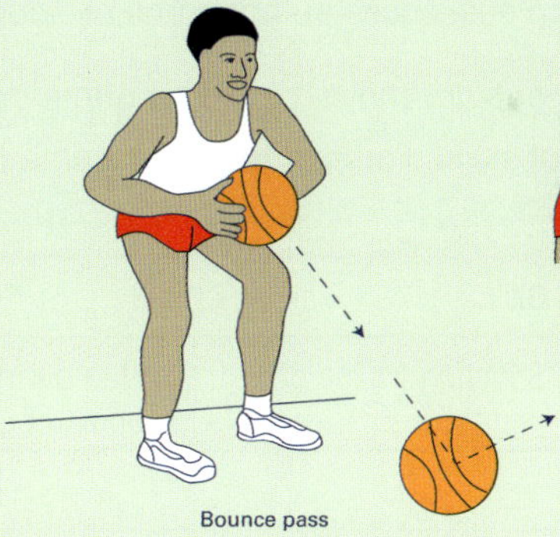

Bounce pass

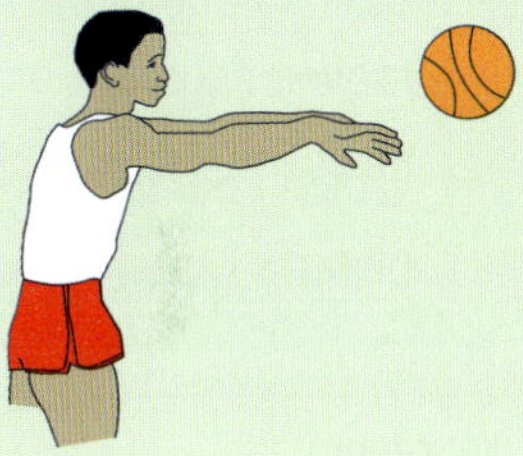

Chest pass

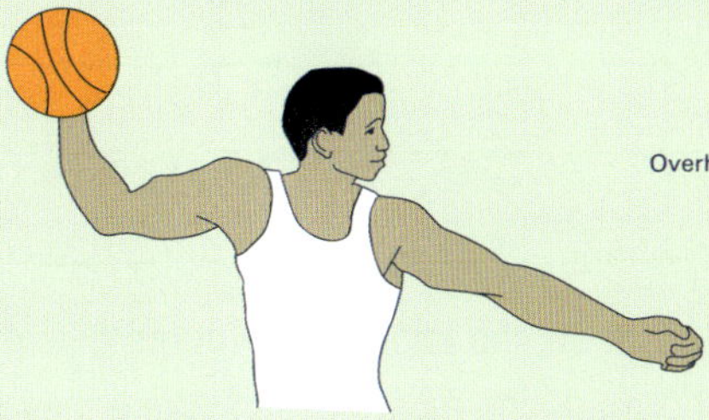

One-handed javelin pass

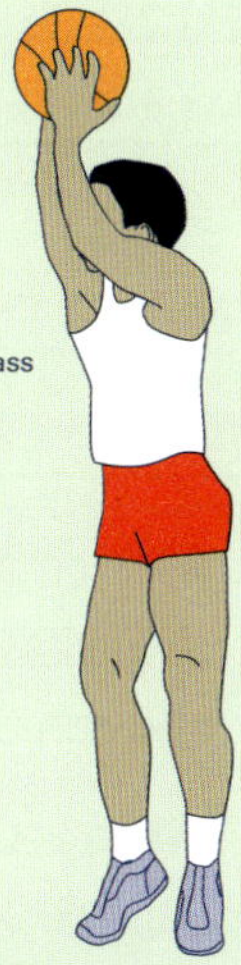

Overhead pass

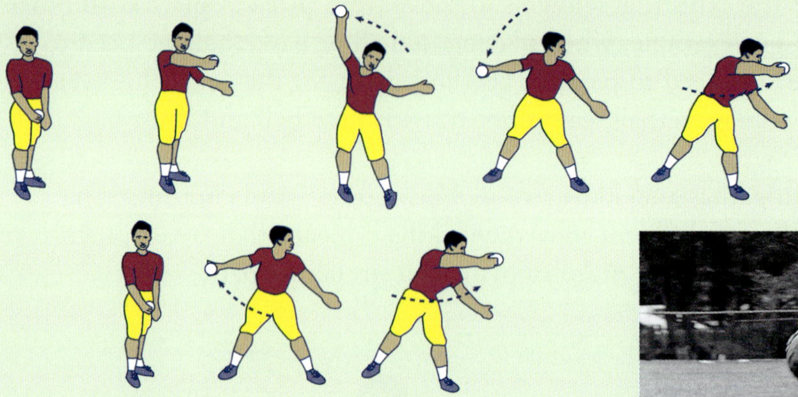

Pitching a softball

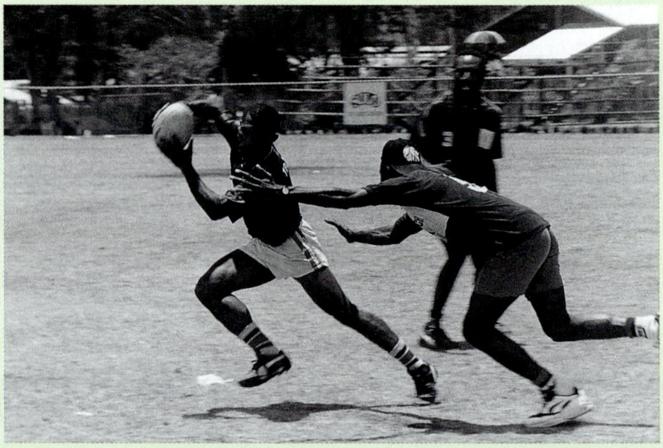

For you to try

- Choose one of the Modified Sports that you like to play. What are your strengths and weaknesses in performing movement skills and sequences in that game or sport?
- Watch your friends or team-mates playing a game against another team and make a tally to show how they perform a number of skills. For example, in a game of basketball or netball you could use a table like this:

Your team	Skill			
	Shooting for the goal	Number of successful shots at goal	Number of passes made	Number of successful passes
Player A				
Player B				
Player C				
Player D				
etc				

After the game work out the total and compare different players. Who made the most shots at goal? Were they successful? Who made the most passes? Were they successful or did the other side get possession of the ball? You can change the table to include different skills for different sports.

- When you are competent at a number of movement skills, how can you maintain your strengths and improve on your weaknesses? Suggest ways to do this.

Keeping fit

PERSONAL FITNESS PROGRAMS

When you are fit you are able to take part in everyday activities without getting tired and able to get your breath back quickly after doing hard physical activity. In order to be physically fit you must exercise regularly. People who follow a traditional way of life are usually fit because they work in the garden, carry water and firewood and walk a lot. In urban areas people often sit down when they are working, ride in cars and buses and use machines like washing machines. The modern way of life may be easier but it is not always healthy, and people in urban areas need to be physically active in order to remain fit and healthy.

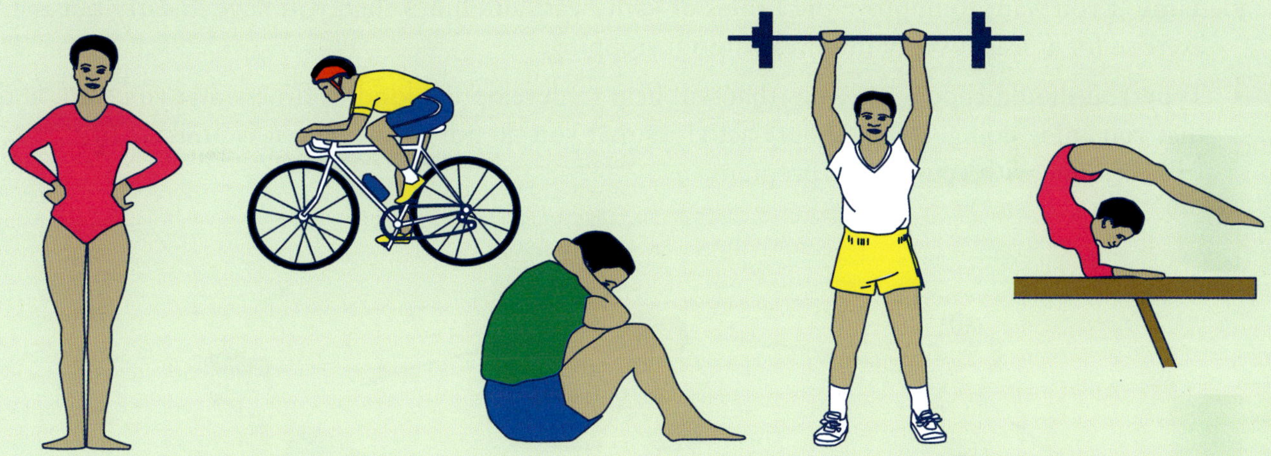

There are different kinds and levels of fitness depending on the activity that you want to do or the sport that you want to play. Fitness is divided into various parts or **components** that include the following:

- muscular strength—the maximum weight that a person can carry
- muscular endurance—how long your muscles can keep going
- stamina or aerobic capacity—how long your lungs can keep going
- speed or anaerobic capacity—how fast you can go for a short time
- flexibility—being able to bend your joints easily when you do different movements
- body composition—how much muscle and fat you have in your body
- balance, agility and coordination.

DESIGNING A FITNESS PROGRAM

You can design a fitness program for yourself and include activities that you enjoy doing and which suit your needs. The four things to remember are *frequency, intensity, time and type*. This is sometimes called the FITT principle.

- **Frequency** Frequency is the number of times that you exercise each week. You should exercise at least three or four times per week if you want to improve your fitness.
- **Intensity** Intensity means how hard the exercise you are doing is, or how hard your heart, muscles and lungs have to work. Walking is good exercise but it does not make your heart and lungs work very hard, so it is called *low-intensity exercise*. Running fast will make your heart and lungs work hard so it is called *high-intensity exercise*. Your heart and breathing rate will increase with the intensity of the exercise because the muscles have to do more work.
- **Time** If you want to improve the fitness of your heart and lungs then you have to carry out the exercise for at least twenty minutes without stopping.
- **Type** You should choose activities that will help to develop the kind of fitness that you want and that you enjoy doing. If you choose activities that you do not enjoy, then it is unlikely that you will continue with your fitness program.

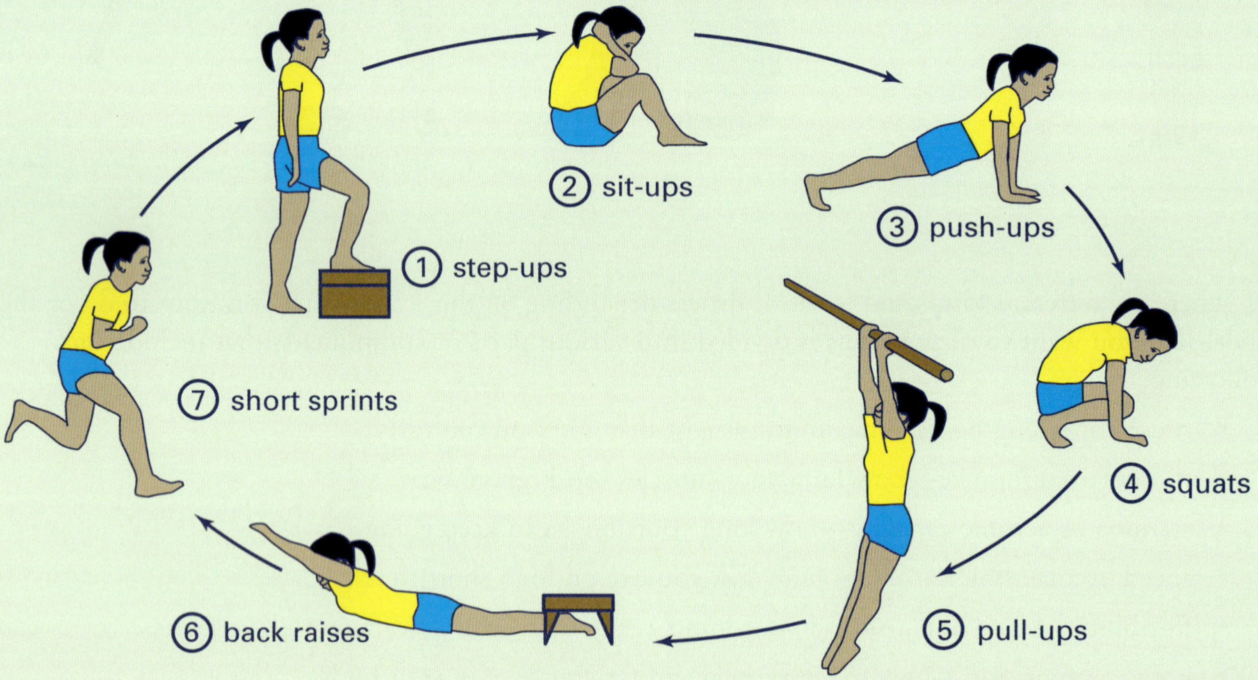

① step-ups
② sit-ups
③ push-ups
④ squats
⑤ pull-ups
⑥ back raises
⑦ short sprints

For you to try

- Make a list of the fitness components that you need to improve and make a program to achieve this.
  — Choose activities that you would like to do to improve each component.
  — Make sure the activities fit in with other things in your life and the time available.
  — Show your rest days.
  — Outline how you will evaluate the program and make changes as required.
  For example:

Fitness components to improve: Muscular endurance and stamina or aerobic capacity			
Day	**Activity**	**Evaluation**	**Changes to be made**
Daily	Walk to school	None	
Monday	Circuit training (7 activities—see diagram on page 92)	Count number of repeats of each activity completed in a given time	Increase number of repeats of each activity as endurance improves.
Tuesday	Rest day		
Wednesday	Run 3 kilometres	Measure time taken	Try to improve time each week. Increase length of run after times stop improving.
Thursday	Rest day		
Friday	Run 3 kilometres	Measure time taken	Try to improve time each week. Increase length of run after times stop improving.
Saturday	Take part in village or school sports competition	None	
Sunday	Rest day		

- Look at the height and weight charts for males and females shown below. Work with a partner to measure and record each other's height and weight. Find your position on the chart. Are you in the healthy range?

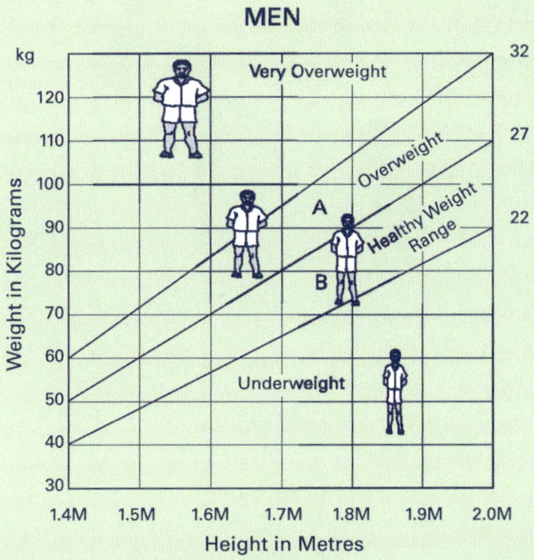

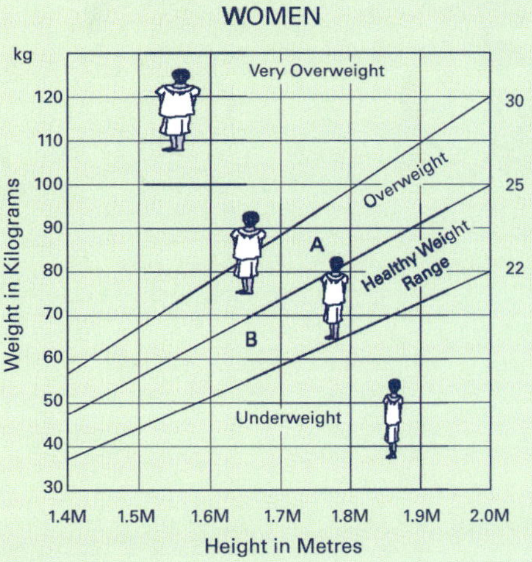

ML SAFETY WHEN PLAYING GAMES AND SPORTS

Whenever we play sport or take part in any game, there is always a risk that we will get an injury or injure somebody else. We need to learn how to avoid those risks that can be avoided and to deal with those risks that cannot be avoided. For example, doing a practice or warm-up activity will help to prevent accidents and injuries.

When people are just playing around, they sometimes like to test the limits just to see how far they can go before something happens. For example, if you are swimming at the beach and playing around in a canoe with your friends, you might see how many people you can get in the canoe. This game would be good fun and you would also learn about how many people can safely sit in the canoe before it sinks, and the way the canoe behaves when it is overloaded. Everybody knows that the canoe will sink and knows that they are going to get wet and have to swim, so they are prepared for the risk. Nobody is likely to get hurt provided everyone can swim and you are close to the beach or the bank of the river.

On the other hand, if you were going to visit friends in another village by canoe, you would not want the canoe to sink and so you would not take the risk of overloading it.

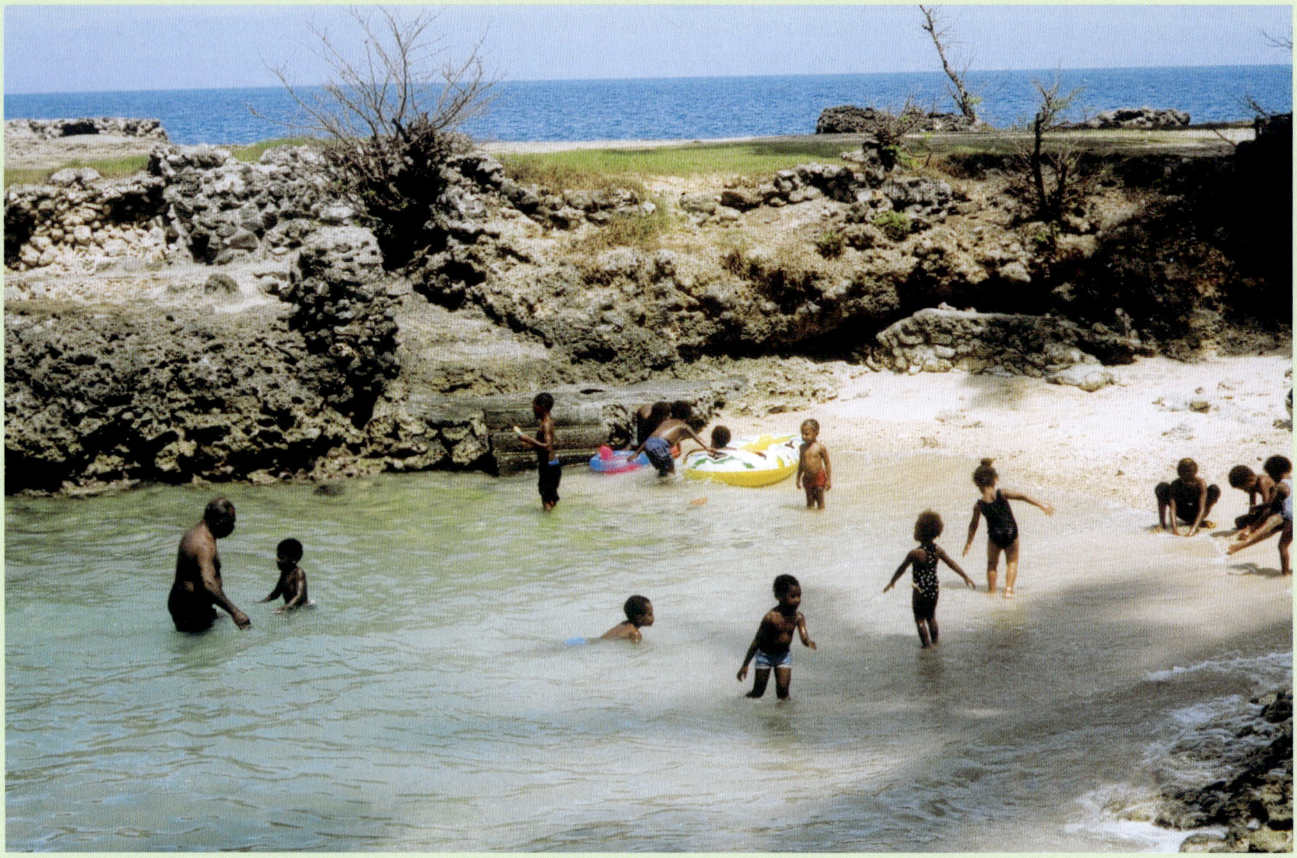

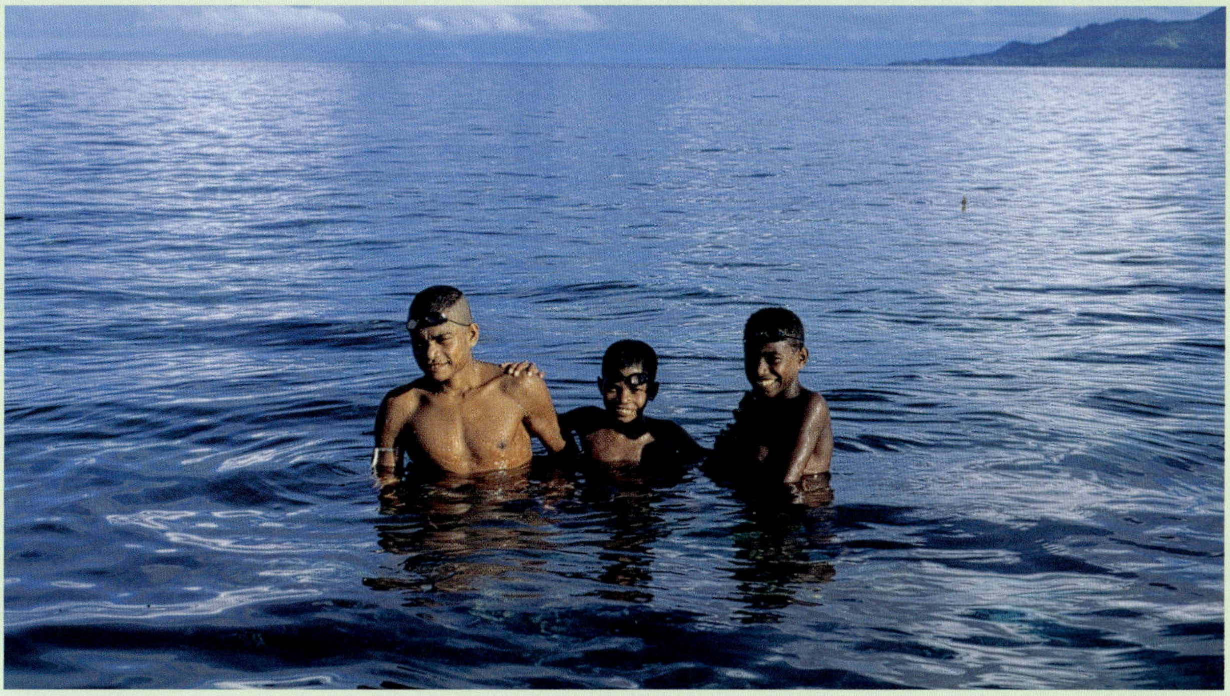

When we assess risk we need to rely on our feelings in order understand the risks involved. Using our feelings in this way is called **instinct** or **gut feeling**. You get a feeling inside that something is not quite right and you then take action to avoid that situation. You need to learn to trust these feelings because they will help you to avoid danger and keep you safe. These feelings are a way of making sure that you stay alive or **survive.**

Sometimes even though we try to avoid risks accidents still happen. We then need to try to learn from the accident. For example, you visit your friends in another village and on the way home the canoe is filled with water. You did not overload the canoe with people, so what happened? Did the weather change and become very rough? Did you carry too much cargo in the canoe? Did it become dark so that you could not see properly? What can you learn from this accident so that you can avoid it in the future?

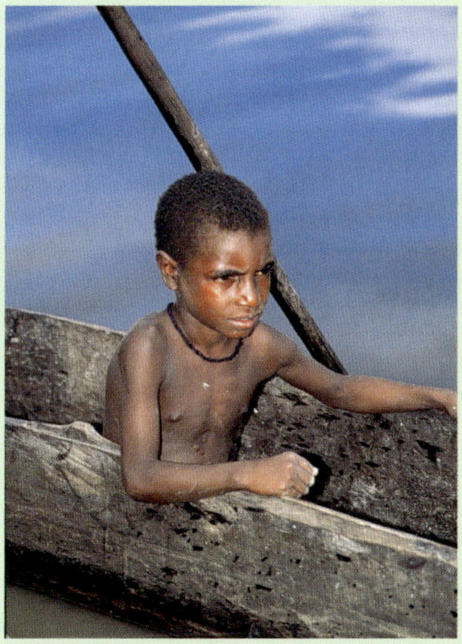

Behaviour that influences safety

There are many things that we can do in order to deal with danger and stay safe:

- seek advice and assistance
- take precautions
- recognise danger signs
- avoid unsafe situations
- carry out safety awareness
- practise injury prevention
- learn first aid

Unsafe behaviour and attitudes

Examples of unsafe behaviour and attitudes are:

- acting without thinking
- showing off or trying to impress your friends by being silly
- rushing in and doing things too quickly or without thinking properly
- refusing to do something that will help to reduce a risk
- being careless and thoughtless
- being aggressive and irresponsible

For you to try

- Make a list of behaviour that can lead to accidents.
- Make groups of four or five students. Think of a situation that you all know something about, such as the example of travelling in a canoe, and list the danger signs that you can think of.
- Think of a situation where something goes wrong, such as an accident, and describe the different ways that you can get help.
- Choose one or two examples of behaviour from the list and carry out a role play to show how they can cause accidents. Show your role play to other members of your class.
- A Make a list of safety tips that people can follow to prevent accidents.

Leisure and recreation

CHOOSING ACTIVITIES ML

Most people enjoy their spare time and the activities that they do in their spare time. Some of these may be individual activities and some may be carried out in groups. It is easier to provide different recreational and leisure activities in a community if there is a recognised need and the community members are interested in helping themselves and supporting the activities.

The choice of recreation and leisure activities that people can take part in depends on a number of factors:

- The type of activities that are available in both rural and urban areas.
- The location of the facilities, and the time and costs involved. Can people easily get to the facilities?
- Whether the activities are available to both males and females. Many facilities are more suited to males than to females.
- The quality of the facilities. Is the equipment complete and working?
- The access that people have. When are the facilities available and how easy is it to use them?

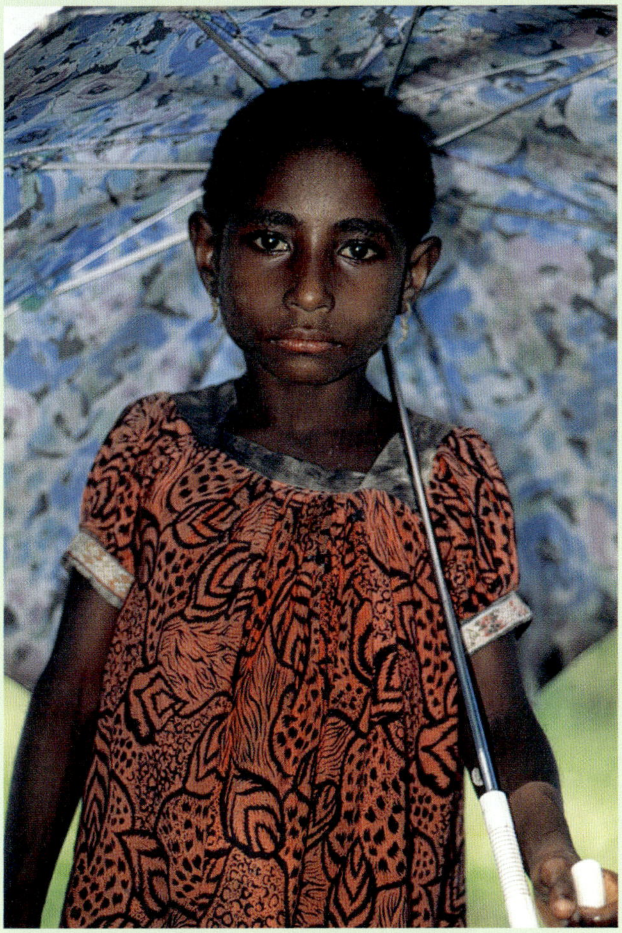

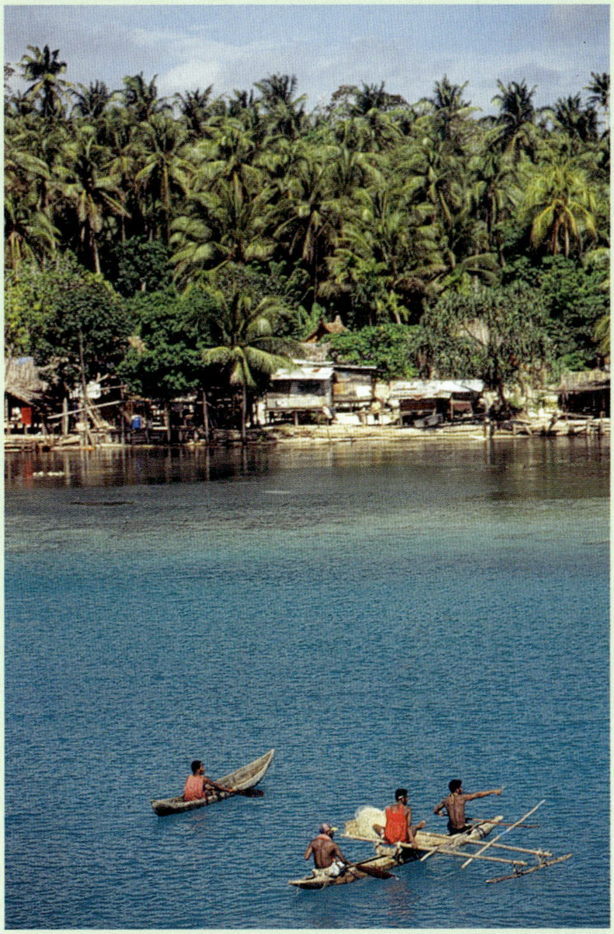

Are activities available to both females and males?

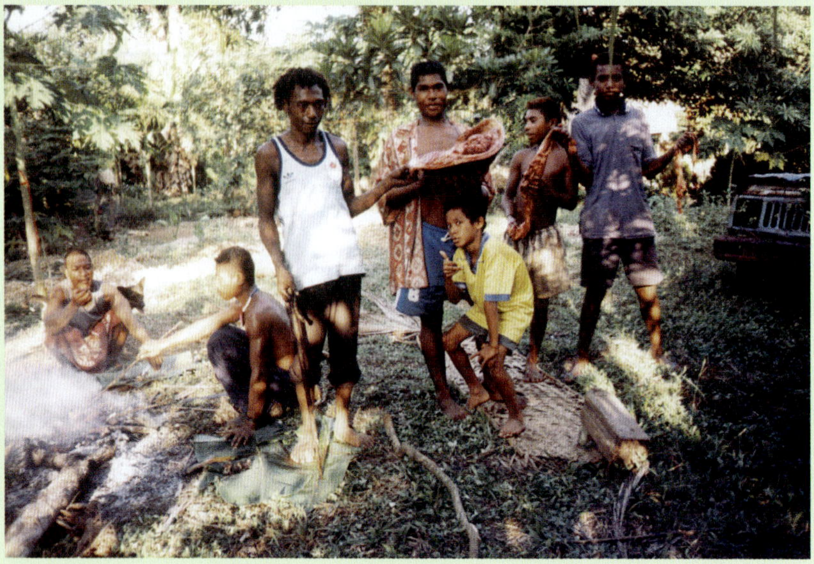

For you to try

- Make a short questionnaire to find out about the recreational activities that people follow in your area or an area that you know well. Think about your questions carefully before you go and interview people. After you have collected the information, make a summary of your results using a simple bar chart. If possible, make a comparison between a rural and an urban area.
- Discuss and list the reasons for the type of recreation and leisure activities that are chosen in your area.
- Suggest a few leisure activities that you would like to see encouraged in a particular area and give your reasons.
- Describe a leisure activity that you would like to see introduced in your area and give reasons. Which group or groups of people would like to take part in this activity? Why would they like to take part?

Sporting roles and responsibilities

WAYS TO COMMUNICATE AND COOPERATE IN TEAM GAMES

Team games are a healthy way to get exercise and enjoy ourselves with other people. Members of a team usually have different skills and abilities, and we need to recognise these differences and learn to make use of them when we play in a competition. For example, in soccer, some players may be better at attacking than defending so we can use this information when we decide what position they will play.

Team games are also important because they teach us to communicate and cooperate with other members of the team. For example, all team games have rules and procedures to follow, and players often need to tell each other about these during the game. Players may also communicate their tactics during the game using words or other signals so that the other team does not know what you are going to do.

If we want to improve in the games and sport that we play or to take part in a competition, then there are certain things that will help us to achieve this:

- Decide what criteria will be used to measure your performance—how do you know how good you are? This does not mean just thinking or feeling that you are the best but deciding what you can measure to find out how good your team is. For example, will you count the points or goals scored? Will you count the number of shots at the goal? Will you measure who has possession of the ball for the greatest time?
- Get feedback, both verbal and non-verbal, from other people who understand the game.
- Practise particular skills and techniques so that you are confident that you can do it well every time.
- Help your team-mates—think and contribute positively and provide feedback to others.
- Learn to recognise different types of behaviour that occur during a match.
- Learn how to help when there is a disagreement during a match or when players are not being treated fairly.

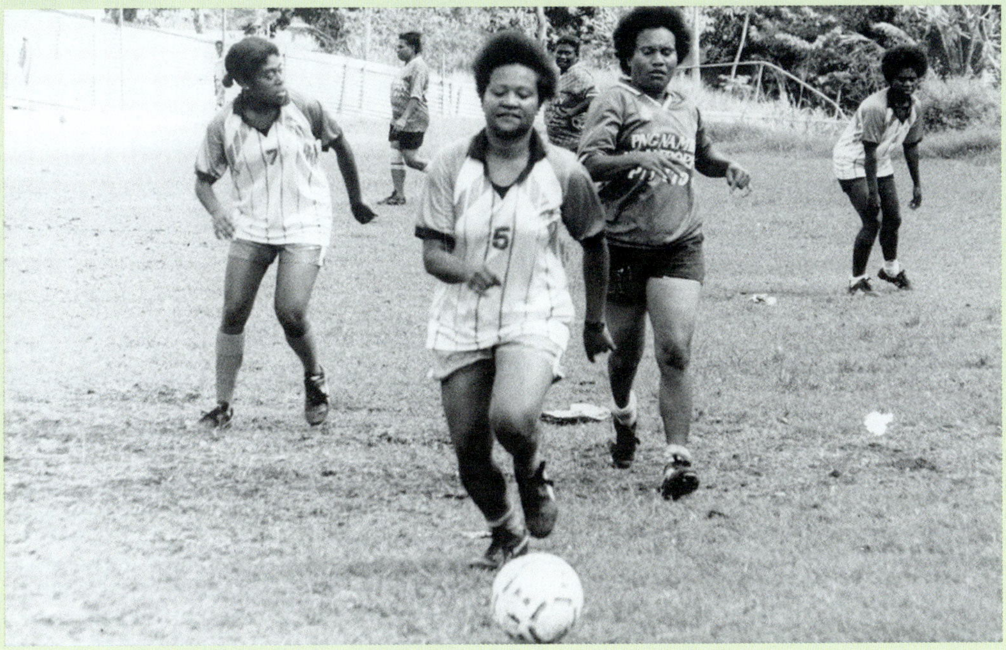

For you to try

- Think of a game or team sport that you play and describe some of the relationships and skills that you have learned in this sport.
- Discuss and list the necessary skills, attitudes and behaviour required to play as a team.
- Describe how to play and communicate more positively during a team game.
- Describe what you will do in order to be able to enjoy a game of sport.

8

Our Culture, Lifestyle and Values

Chapter Summary

In this chapter you will have an opportunity to:

- ✔ Find out about traditional cultures and practices that contribute to our national identity
- ✔ Find out about different lifestyles and the choices that we can make in the way that we live

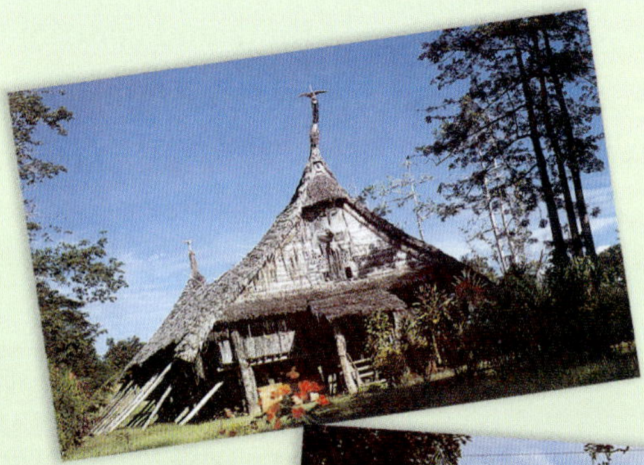

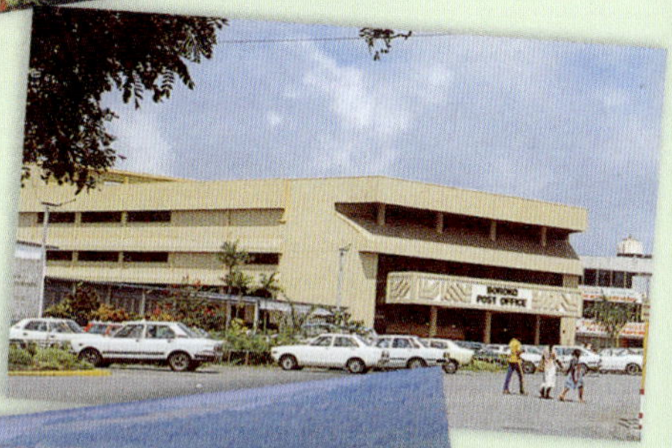

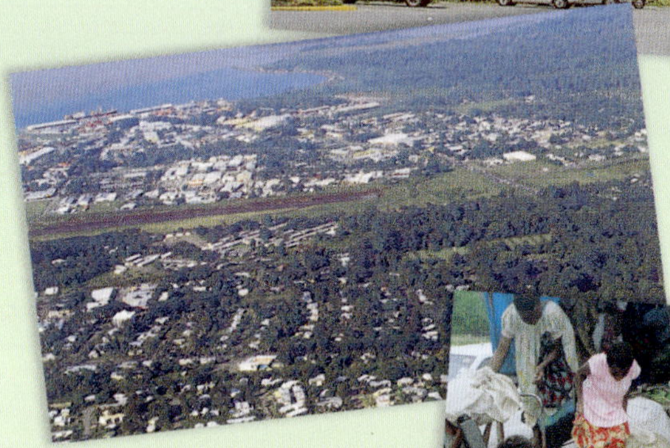

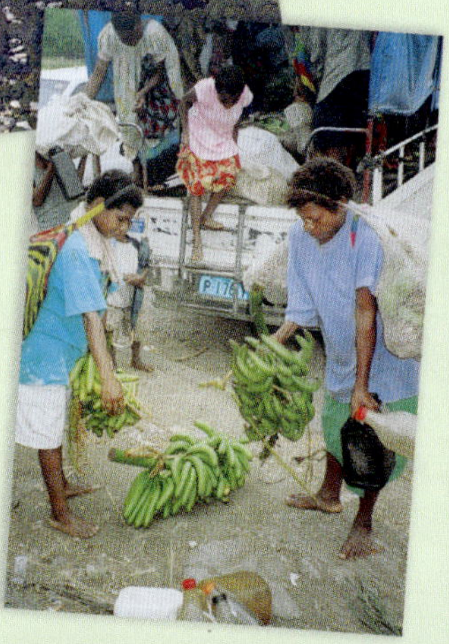

Syllabus references

Strand: Our culture, lifestyle and values
Sub-strands: Culture and values, lifestyle changes

Outcomes:

8.3.1 Consider how traditional cultures and customs contribute to national identity

8.3.2 Compare a range of lifestyles and outline elements of a lifestyle they would prefer in the future

Culture and values

TRADITIONAL CULTURES AND CUSTOMS ML

Key facts

- Traditional cultures and customs are an important part of our national identity in Papua New Guinea.
- We show our national identity through symbols such as the flag, the national emblem, the national anthem, our currency, the parliament and national animals and plants.
- There is a range of different lifestyles such as village life, town life, and city or suburban life.
- Each lifestyle is different because of its elements or parts such as type of housing, diet and type of services available.
- We can choose the type of lifestyle that we would like to live, although there are advantages and disadvantages to every lifestyle.

In Papua New Guinea, traditional cultures and customs are still strong and are an important part of the people's way of life, especially for those living in rural areas. In many countries the traditions have been lost, so when visitors come to Papua New Guinea they enjoy being able to see the culture of the people in different areas.

Language is an important part of the culture and Papua New Guinea is famous for having so many different local languages—about 860 altogether. The three languages that are most commonly spoken are English, Pidgin and Motu, and Members of Parliament may use any of these three. Many Papua New Guineans can speak several languages, and when people are away from their own area, they often like to meet with their wantoks who can speak the same language.

Traditional dress and traditional dancing continue to be important, and most people in Papua New Guinea know dances from their own area. Students in schools often learn dances from other students and teachers from other provinces and perform these on special occasions. Visitors from other countries quickly learn to recognise Asaro mudmen, Western Highlands dancers or the tapioca dance from the Trobriand Islands.

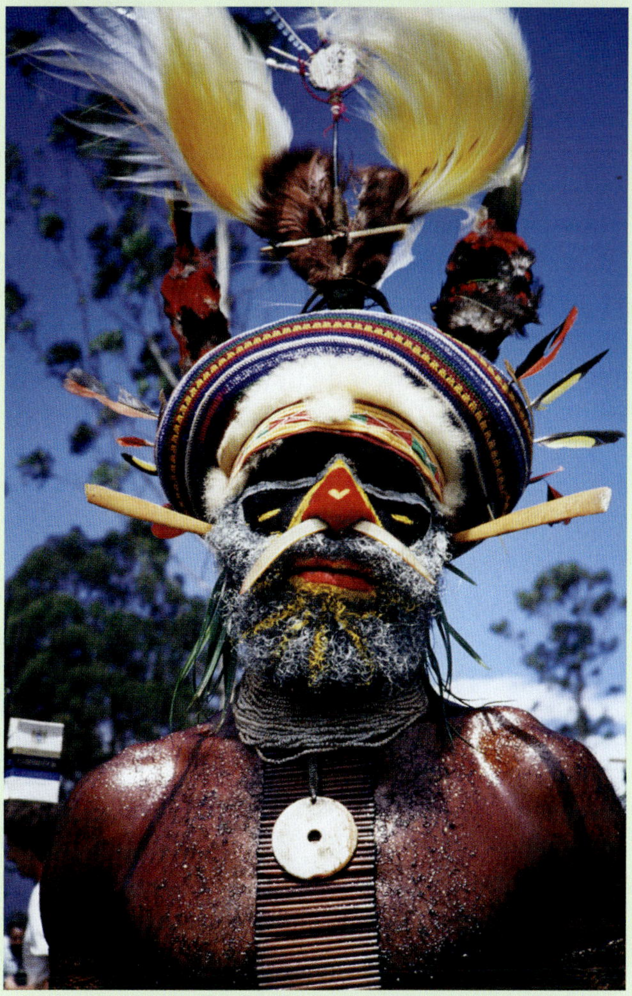

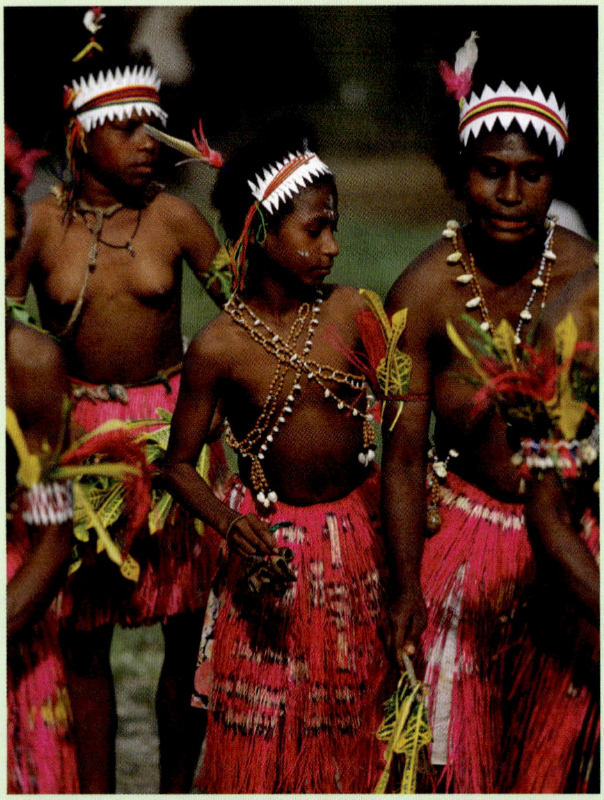

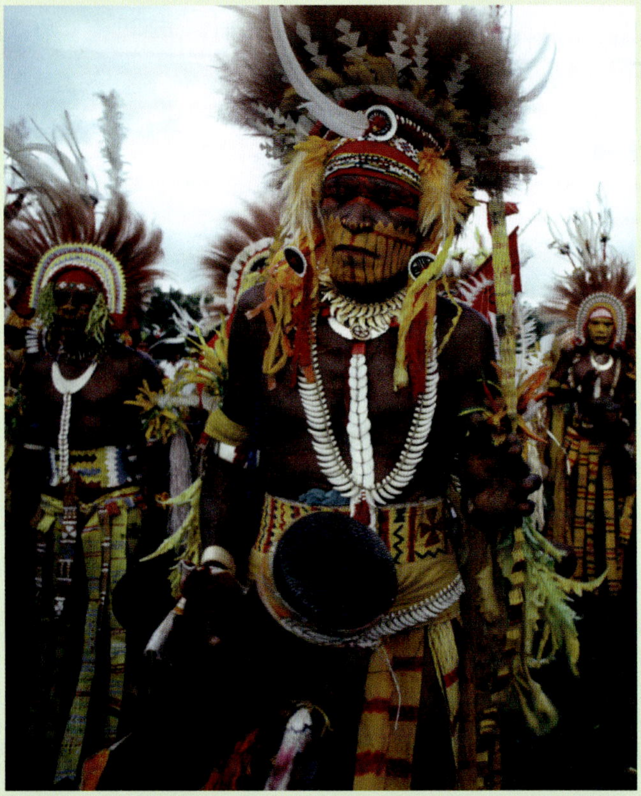

Even though rice is now found in almost every part of Papua New Guinea, many people still grow and enjoy their traditional staple food. For example, in parts of the Markham Valley, people cook bananas every day; in parts of Western Province making sago is important; and in the Highland provinces and elsewhere sweet potato is the staple food.

The way that people build houses also varies a lot in different parts of the country. On the coast, traditional houses are usually raised off the ground on posts or stumps and have windows or shutters and sometimes more than one door. Making the house higher and having windows and doors helps the breeze to move through the house and keep it cooler. A house that sits on posts also gives an area under the house that can be used for sitting, storing firewood or drying clothes. In the Highlands, traditional houses are usually on the ground, round in shape and have only one door and no windows. This way of

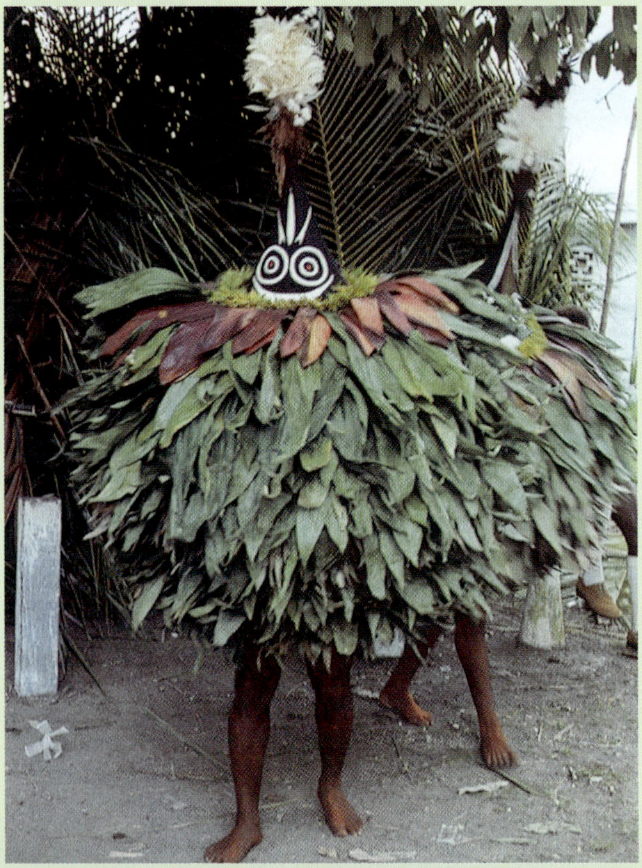

building helps to keep the house warm, especially at night. In the Sepik the people build a **haus tambaran** that is only found in this part of Papua New Guinea.

Different styles of building from different provinces can be seen in the National Parliament buildings in Port Moresby. For example, the front of the main building is like a haus tambaran and the part of the building that is used by Members of Parliament is designed like a highlands roundhouse.

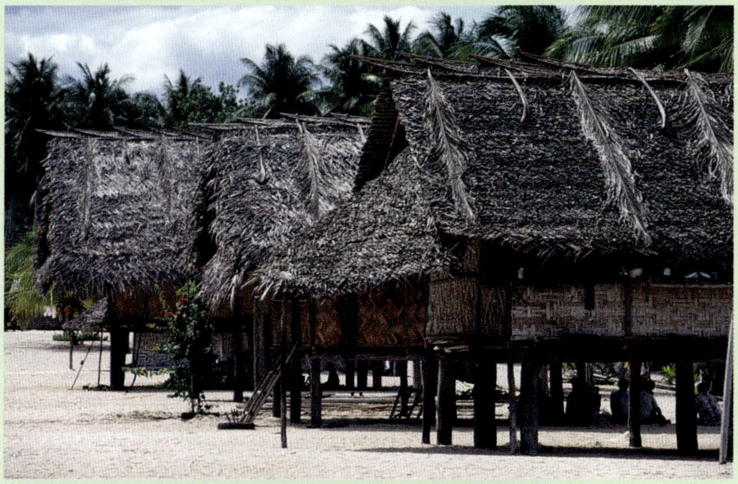

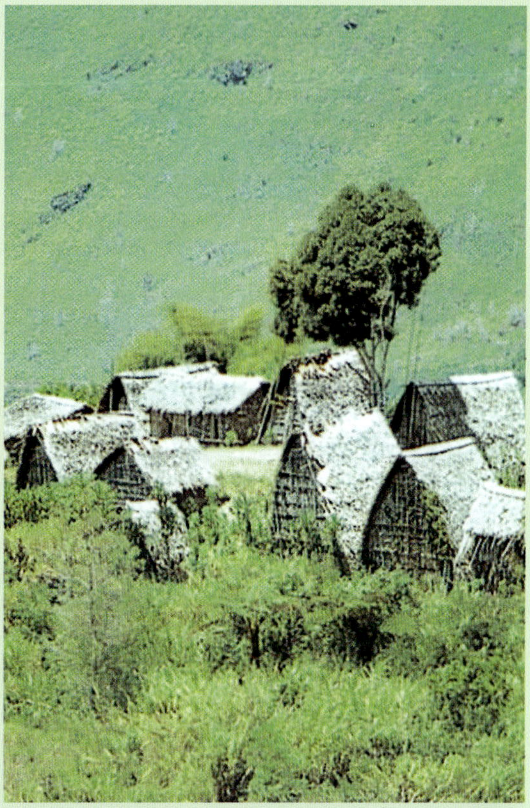

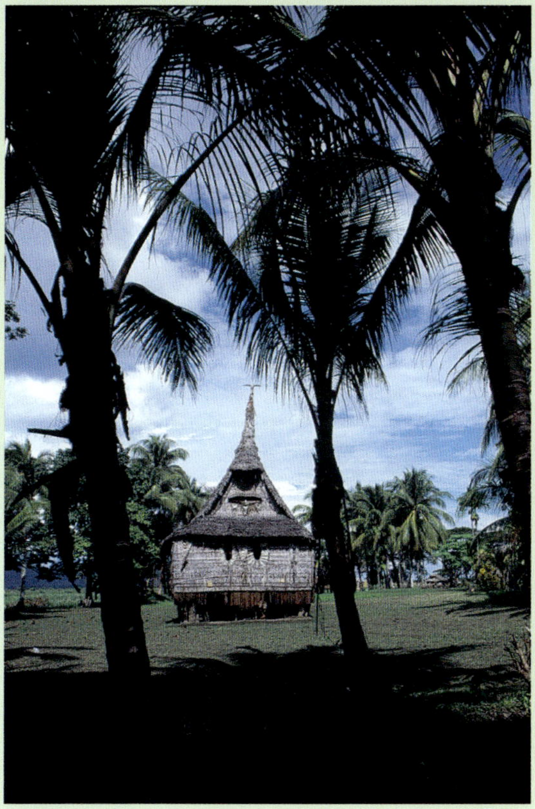

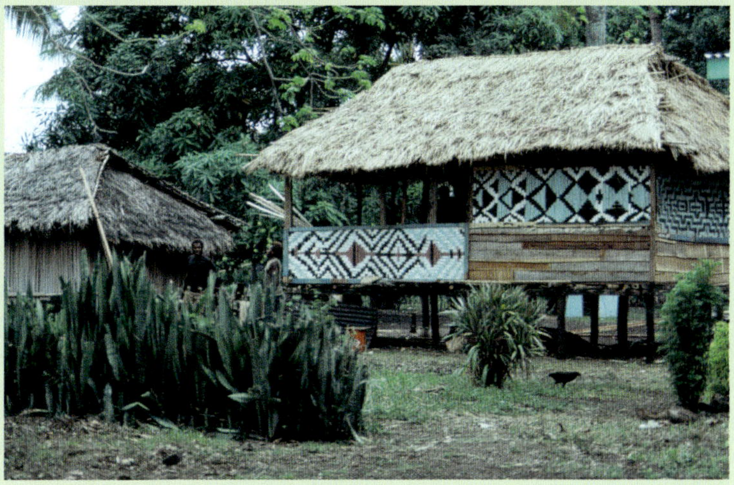

Traditional trading and traditional money continue to be important in many parts of Papua New Guinea. For example, the people living in the islands of Milne Bay exchange shell necklaces called **bagi** and armlets with each other as part of the **kula**. The necklaces move in one direction around the ring and the armlets move in the opposite direction. In the New Guinea Islands, tabu shell money is still used during traditional ceremonies. In the Highlands, kina shells are worn during traditional dancing and exchanged during important ceremonies.

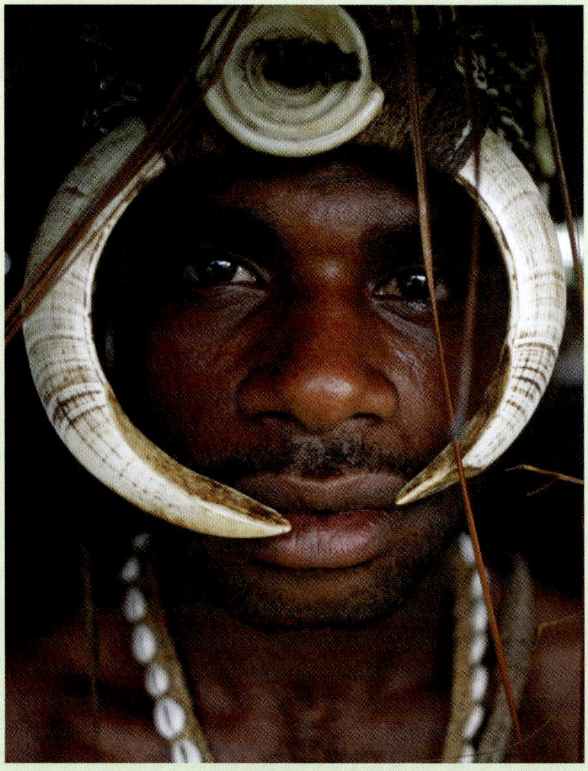

People living in the rural areas carry out their own customs according to their own timetable. These customs are sometimes associated with the seasons, with planting and harvesting of food crops or with other important occasions in the community such as weddings and funerals. In more urban areas these celebrations usually happen during national days such as Independence Anniversary, although people from a particular place who are living in a town may get together to make a celebration for a particular reason.

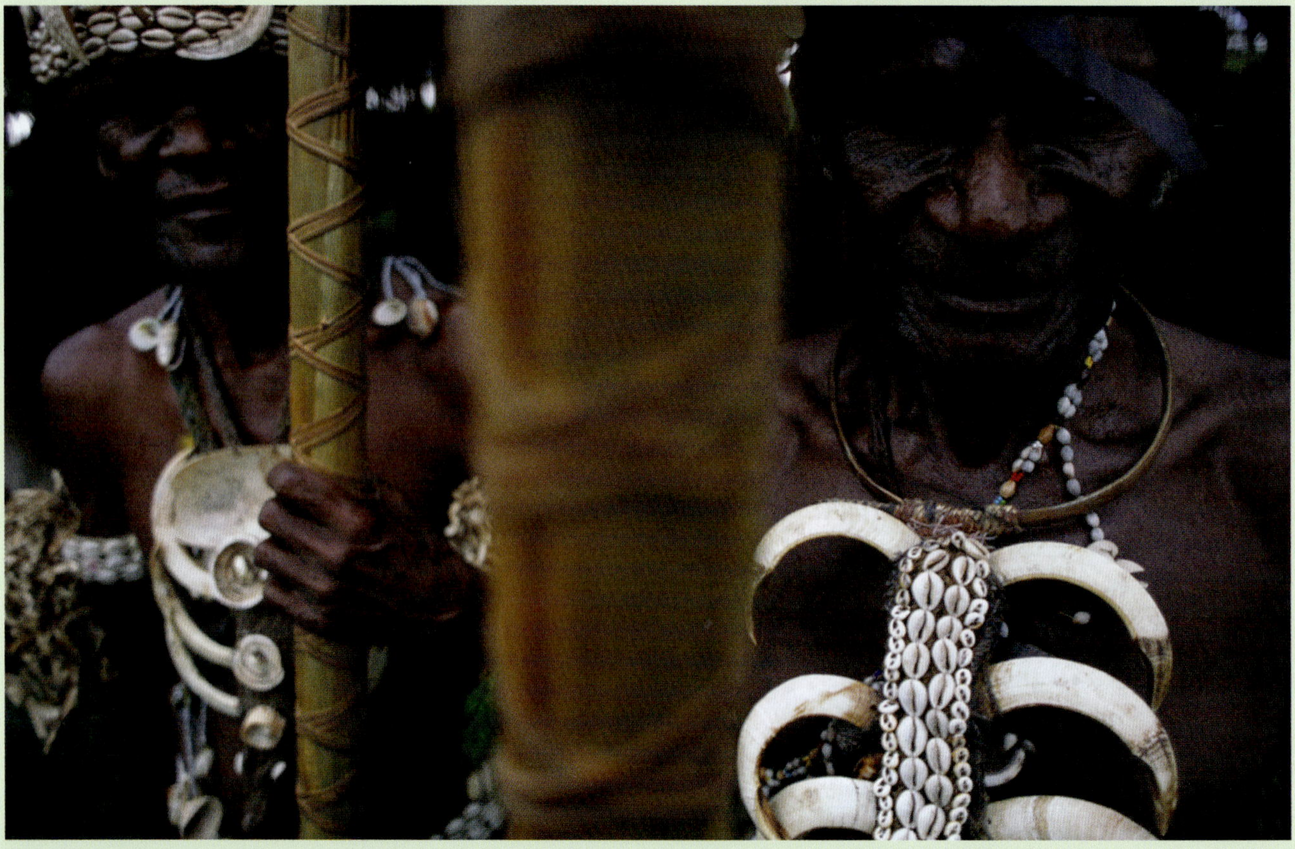

NATIONAL IDENTITY

We show our national identity in Papua New Guinea in a number of ways.

- The national flag, which was designed by a student from Yule Island. One half shows a yellow bird of paradise on a red background and represents Papua New Guinea moving into nationhood. The other half shows stars known as the Southern Cross, which is only seen in the night skies of the southern hemisphere.

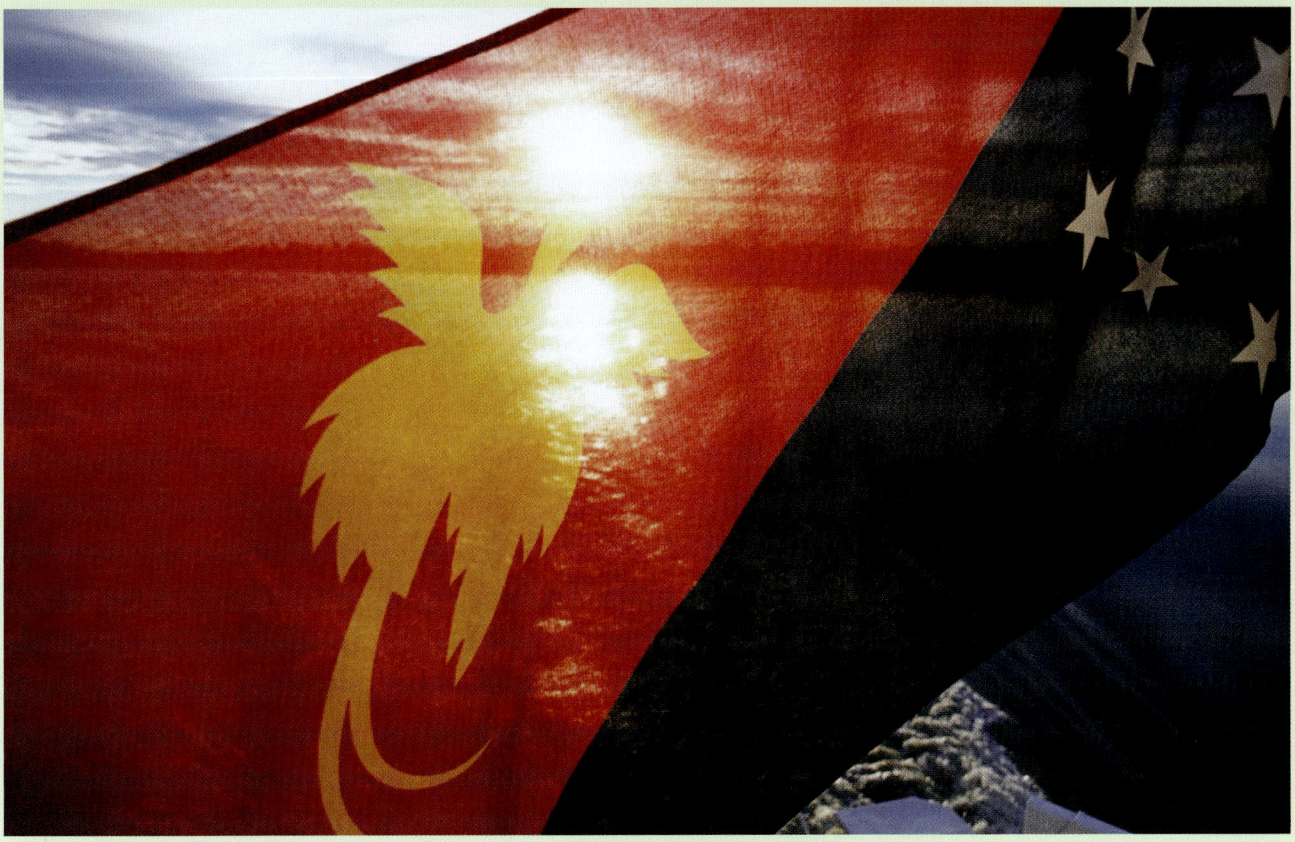

- The national emblem, which shows a kundu drum and spear together with a bird of paradise with wings outstretched. All three of these are found in many parts of the country. The emblem can only be used for official government purposes and is found on the front of the Papua New Guinea passport.

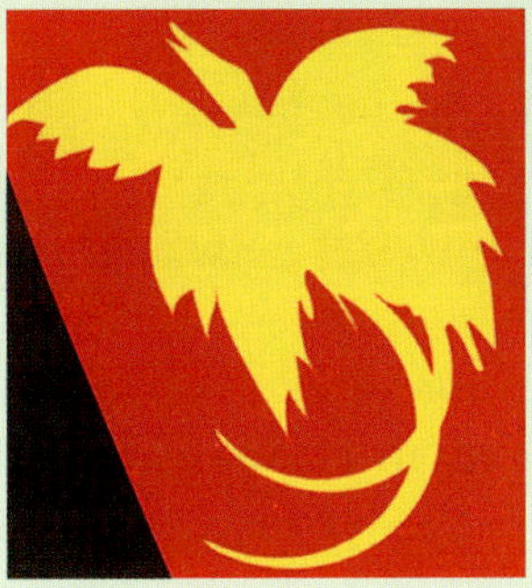

- The national currency, kina and toea, are named after two types of shell money. Traditionally, the kina shell is often worn around the neck and the toea shells on the arms.

- Parliament Haus includes building styles from different parts of Papua New Guinea and also includes carving and painting from different provinces. Block A, the main building, is designed in the style of a Sepik haus tambaran, and block C is designed in the style of a Highlands' roundhouse.
  - — The water around the main building represents the importance of the sea to Papua New Guinea.
  - — Above the main entrance of the Grand Hall, nineteen ancestral masks, one from each province, are carved in kwila under the mosaic.
  - — The garamut drum, which calls people together, is carved into the front of the Speaker's desk as a symbol of the work of the Speaker.

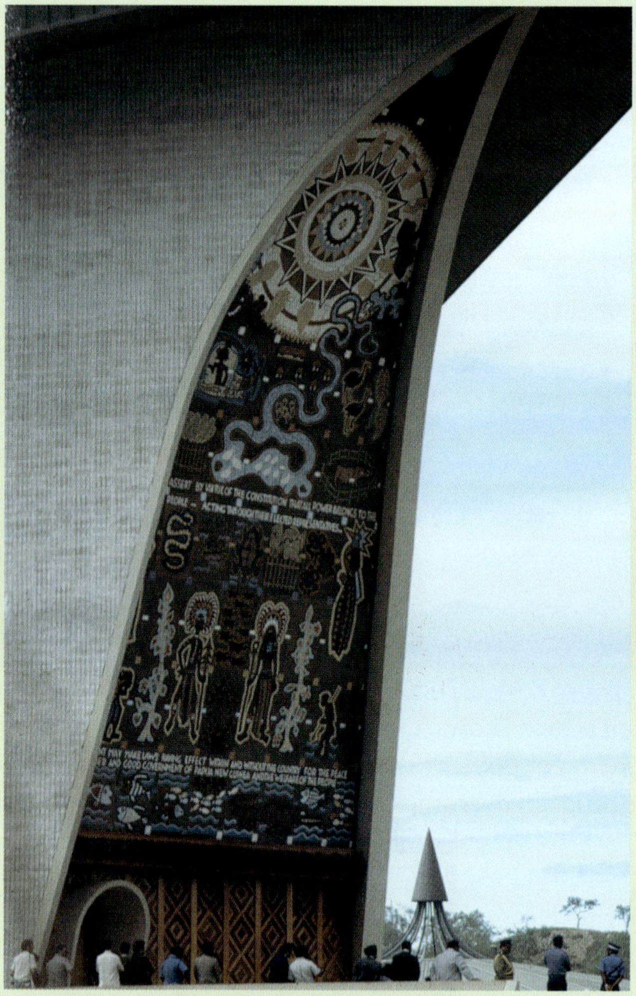

- Many of the special animals and plants in Papua New Guinea are shown on coins and stamps. Many of these animals are found only in PNG, such as the bird of paradise, cuscus and certain butterflies.
- The national song, which is played and sung on important occasions and at the beginning of important sporting events. It was first played at the Olympic Games in Montreal, Canada, in 1976.

O arise all you sons

O arise all you sons of this land,
Let us sing of our joy to be free;
Praising God and rejoicing to be
Papua New Guinea.

Shout our name from the mountains to sea,
Papua New Guinea;
Let us raise our voices and proclaim,
Papua New Guinea.

Now give thanks to the good Lord above
For His kindness, His goodness and love,
For this land of our fathers so free
Papua New Guinea.

Shout again for the whole world to hear
Papua New Guinea.
We're independent and we're free,
Papua New Guinea.

For you to try

- Make some coin rubbings of the animals that are shown on different coins. You can do this by putting the coin under a piece of paper and carefully rubbing over it with a soft pencil. It is best to hold the pencil so that it is almost parallel to the paper.
- Make a list of the animals that are shown on the coins and notes of Papua New Guinea and classify these animals into groups.
- Find out about those parts of the culture that are common to people from different regions. Make a list of those parts that are common.
- Give a two-minute talk to the class to describe how parts of local cultures contribute to national identity.
- Make a group of four or five students and discuss the following: How do we show pride in different parts of our culture? What values are shown by these feelings?
- Make a group of four or five students and discuss the following: Should one of the three national languages ever become the only national language? What are the advantages and disadvantages of this happening?

Lifestyle and changes SS ML

VILLAGE, TOWN AND CITY

The way that people choose to live is known as their **lifestyle**. People in Papua New Guinea live different kinds of lifestyle depending on the place where they live and other circumstances.

For example, many people still live a village way of life, which they have done for thousands of years. They grow their own food and go fishing, and may go hunting. Many people also keep chickens and pigs to improve their diet. They make their own houses from bush materials, although bush material houses have to be replaced regularly as they get old and rotten. People are also now using modern building materials to make houses in the village. These houses cost more money but last longer, and a corrugated iron roof can be used to collect rainwater in a tank. This is useful because there may be no water supply in the village. Other services may be missing from the village as well, such as electricity or telephone. There may also be no roads or reliable transport.

Town life is different, although not all towns are the same. Most people in towns live in houses built from modern materials, and there is usually a water supply, a sewerage system for waste (with flush toilets), electricity and other services like telephones and transport that help to improve the quality of life. People living in towns may have a small garden but need to buy most of their food from the market and the store, so their diet is limited by what is available and what they can afford. People living in towns need to earn money to pay for their food and the services that they use.

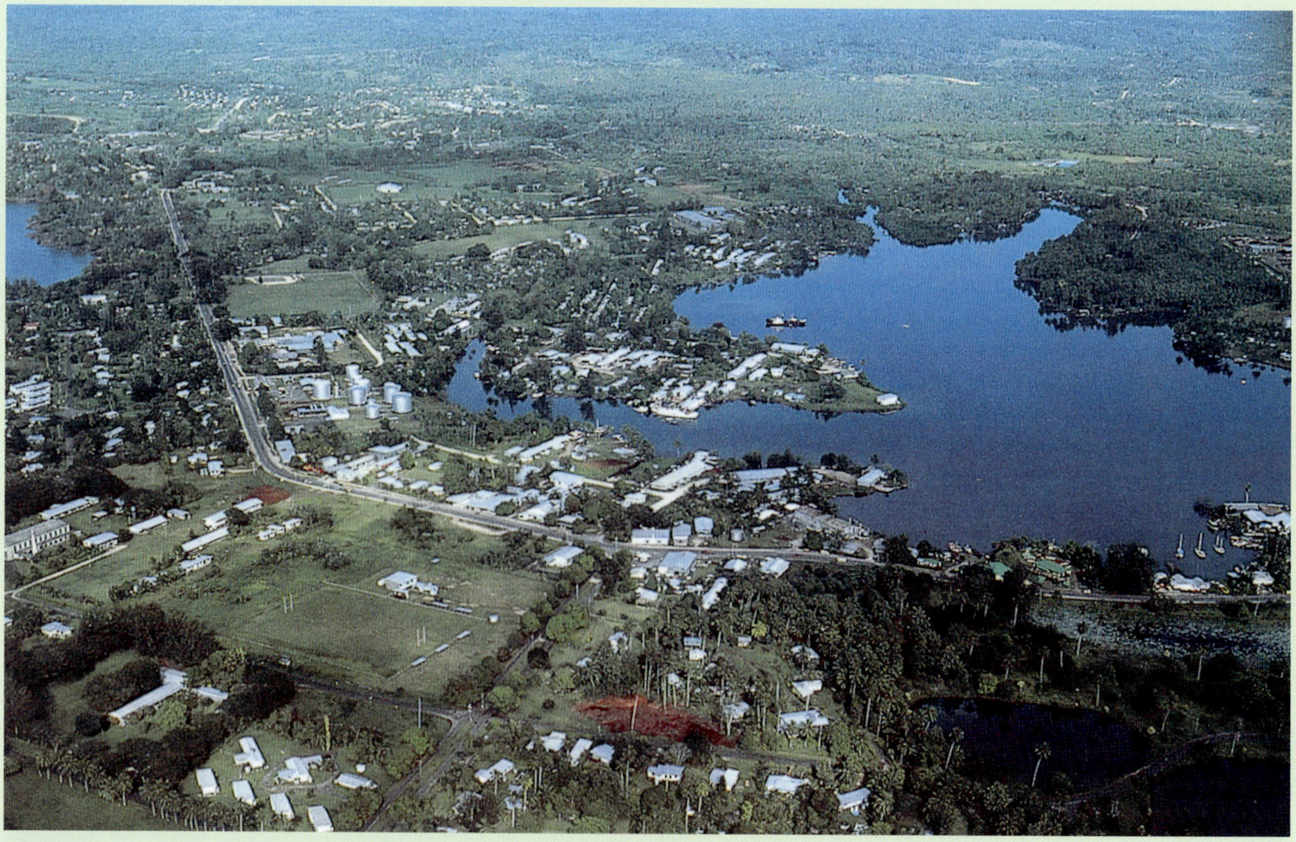

Madang

Cities like Port Moresby are divided into different areas called **suburbs.** Cities can have better houses and services than towns and villages, but many people cannot afford to pay for these because they are very expensive. Although there is a water supply and electricity, there are still times when these break down. Living in a town or city without reliable water is very difficult.

Some people want to go and live in towns but do not have a job or house, so they build squatter settlements or shanty towns on the outskirts of the town. They do not have enough land to grow food, and unless they can find a job they may not have enough money to buy food. There may be no river or well for water and there is no town water supply. There is usually not enough firewood, so they may cut down the trees planted by the council to make the town look attractive.

People in squatter settlements are trying to live a village lifestyle in the town or city, but this is not suitable and so the way of life is very hard. The squatter lifestyle has the disadvantages of both the village and town ways of life with few of the advantages.

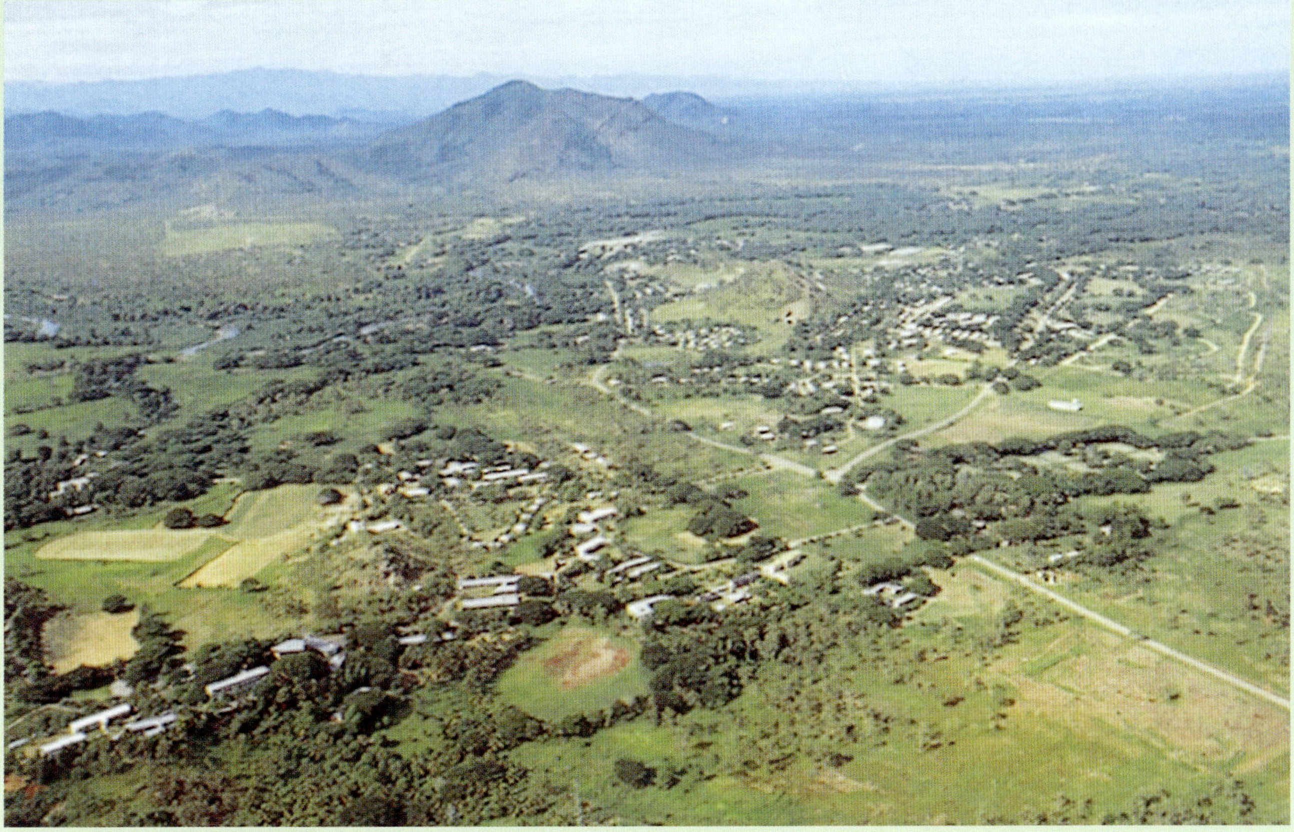

Outer suburbs of Port Moresby

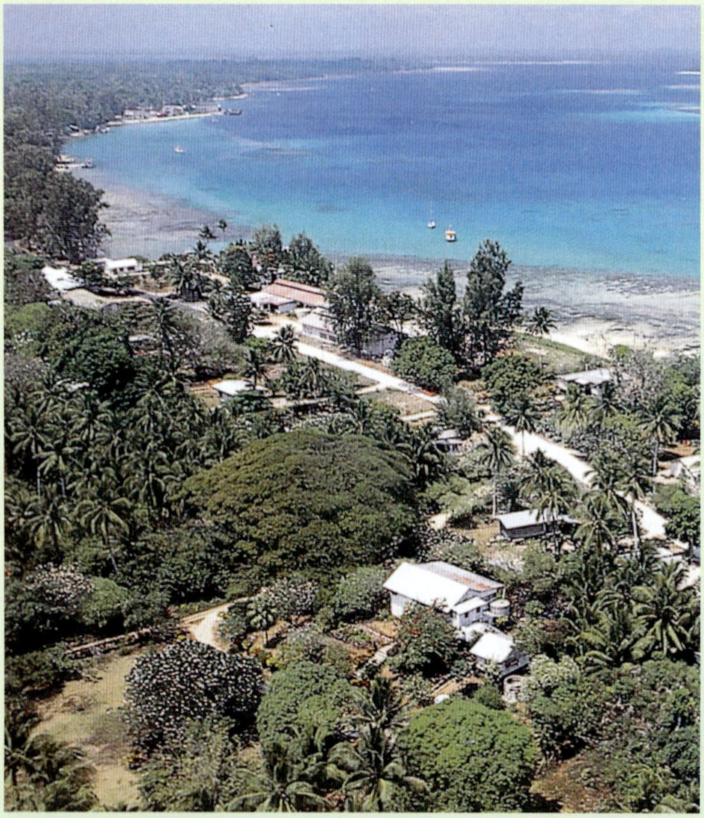

Kavieng, New Ireland

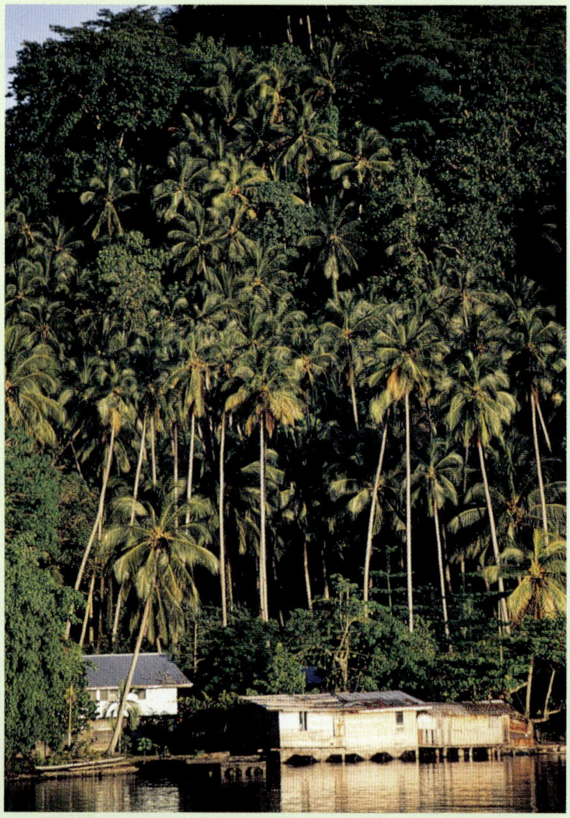

Witu Islands

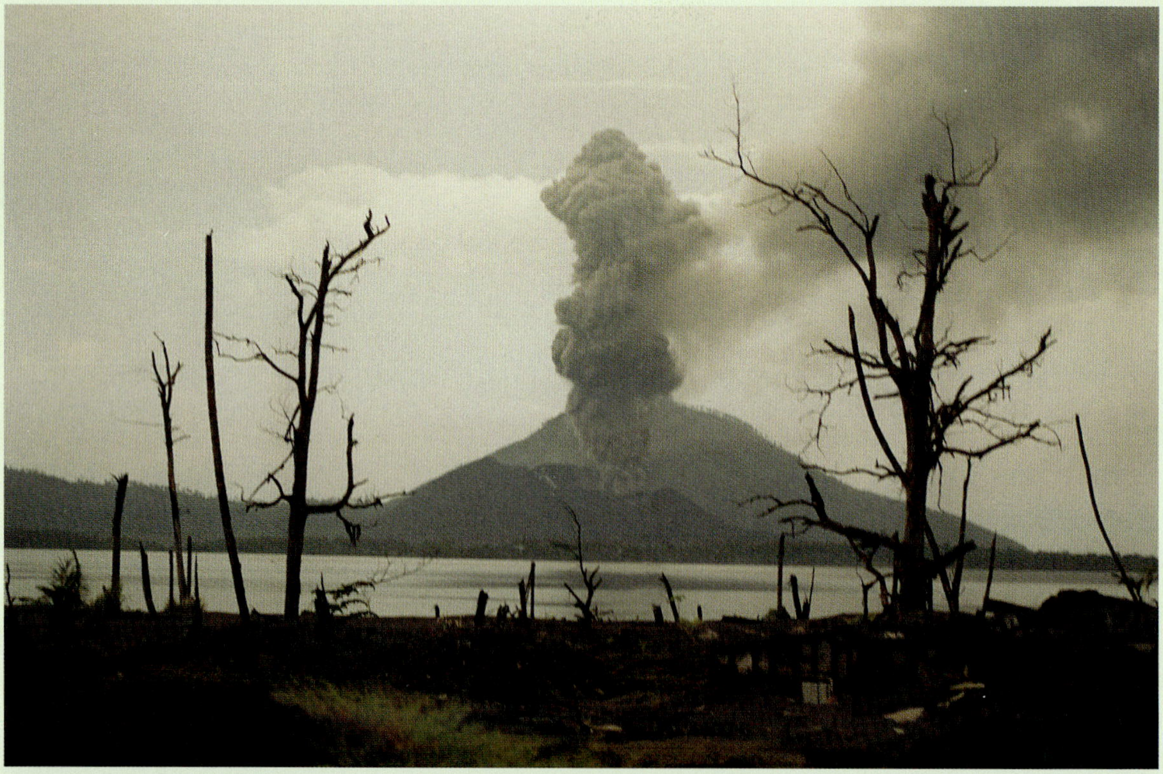

Rabaul after the volcanic eruption

REASONS FOR CHOOSING DIFFERENT LIFESTYLES (ML)

People have different reasons for choosing the place where they live and the way that they live. For example:

- to get an education
- to find employment
- to be able to travel and see different places
- to enjoy a traditional way of life and be part of a community

After living and working in towns for many years, many Papua New Guineans are now building houses back in the village and going to live there. After living away for many years they can see the advantages of a village lifestyle and want to return to live in the community in which they grew up.

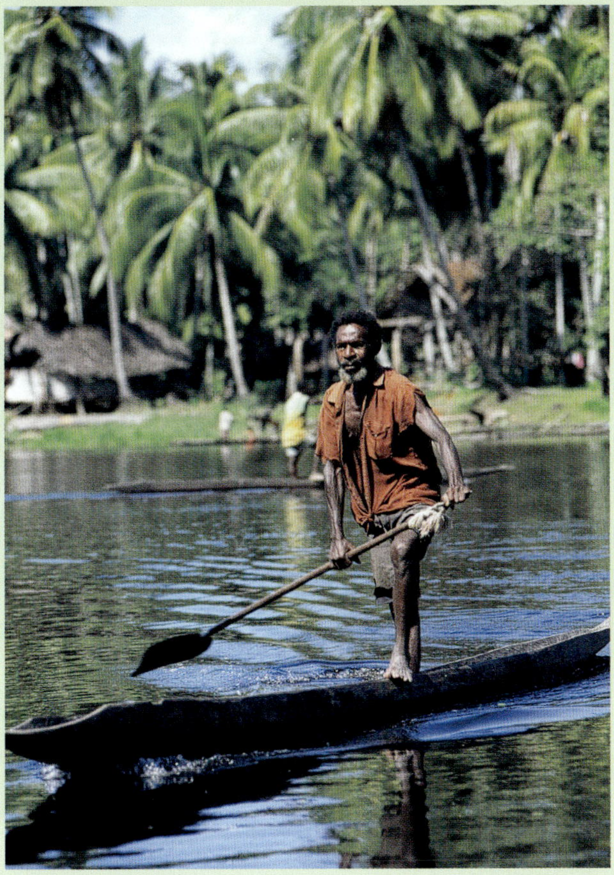

For you to try

- Find out more about different kinds of lifestyle. Describe some of the different parts of these lifestyles.
- What opportunities and choices are available to you in your lifestyle? Describe the choices.
- A Choose a lifestyle that you would like to follow. Give reasons for choosing it and describe how you will achieve the goals of your lifestyle.

9

Health of Individuals and Population

Chapter Summary

In this chapter you will have an opportunity to:

- ✔ Find out about different behaviour that promotes growth and development
- ✔ Find out about the differences that occur in our growth and development and the ways that we can deal with those differences
- ✔ Find out about different beliefs and values about sexuality
- ✔ Find out about different reasons that people have for choosing food
- ✔ Make a plan to deal with a nutrition-related issue in your school and carry out the plan
- ✔ Find out about the health issues that are important to young people and work out health goals
- ✔ Find out about safe sexual behaviour and sexual responsibilities
- ✔ Learn ways to deal with unsafe or risky situations
- ✔ Learn to identify a community health concern and how to respond to that concern
- ✔ Find out more about the effects of growth in family size and the community and how this affects health services and community facilities
- ✔ Find out more about the effect of using drugs in the community
- ✔ Find out about the support provided by different groups in the community to help people deal with drugs

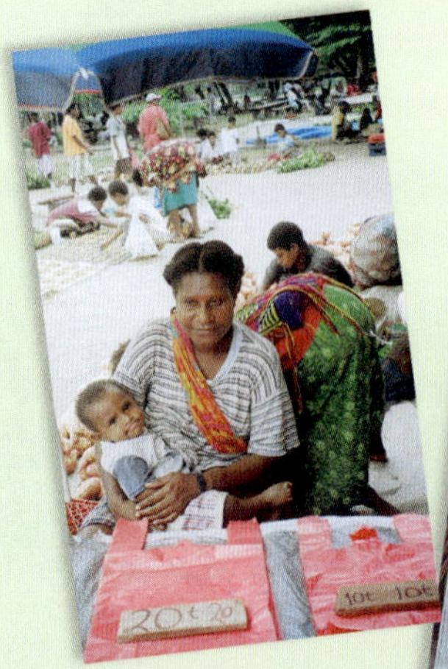

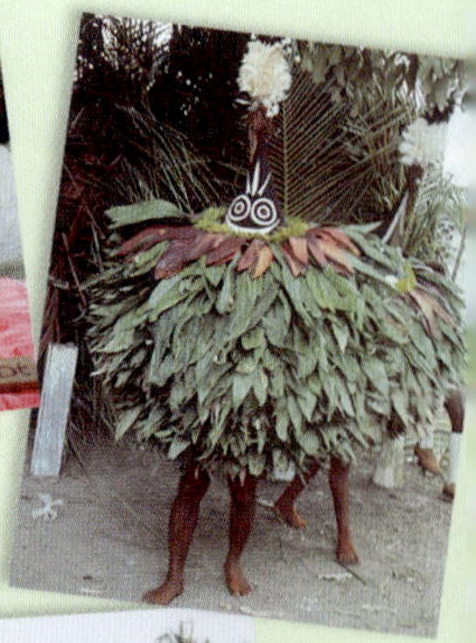

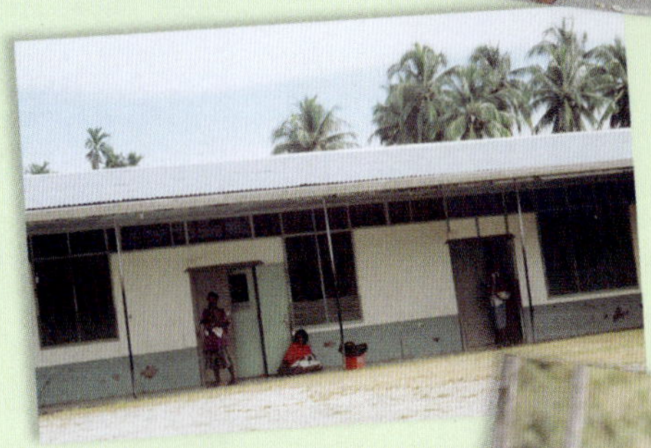

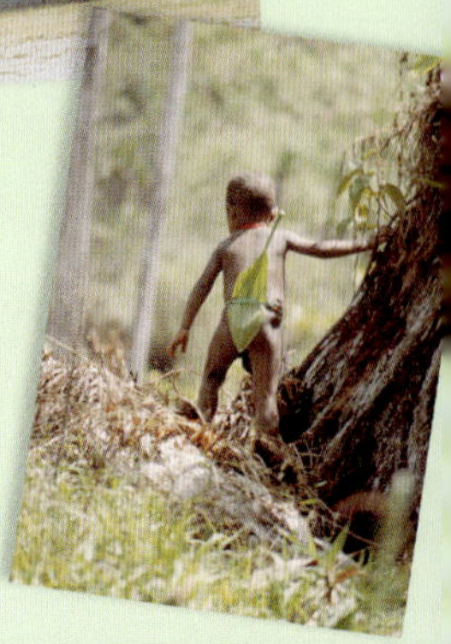

Syllabus references

Strand: Health of individuals and population
Sub-strands: Growth and development, nutrition, personal health and safety, community health, use of drugs

Outcomes:

- **8.4.1** Identify and describe the behaviour that promotes growth and development, taking into account heredity and environment
- **8.4.2** Outline issues arising from differences in rates of growth and development and how individuals manage the changes
- **8.4.3** Identify different cultural beliefs and values about sexuality
- **8.4.4** Discuss some social, physiological, cultural and environmental reasons for people's food choices
- **8.4.5** Plan, develop and implement strategies to address a nutrition-related issue in the school
- **8.4.6** Outline health issues that are of concern to young people
- **8.4.7** Discuss safe sexual behaviour and sexual responsibilities
- **8.4.8** Develop strategies to respond to unsafe or risky situations
- **8.4.9** Identify a community health concern and propose actions to respond to that concern
- **8.4.10** Describe the effects of family size and growing communities on the provision of health services and community facilities
- **8.4.11** Evaluate the effects of drug use on the community
- **8.4.12** Describe the programs offered by support agencies and counselling programs in the community

Key facts

- In order to grow and develop properly, we must follow certain types of behaviour such as eating properly, taking exercise, keeping clean and avoiding drugs.
- Young people grow and develop at different speeds and we need to learn to deal with these differences.
- As we grow up, our sexuality develops and we learn to think, feel and behave as a man or woman. There are different cultural beliefs and values about sexuality.
- Eating is a behaviour that varies between people from different places. People eat different kinds of food for different reasons.
- When an issue related to diet or nutrition arises, we need to make a plan in order to deal with that issue.
- Young people have particular health issues that are related to their position in the community.
- One health issue facing young people comes from sexual behaviour. We need to learn safe sexual behaviour and to be responsible.
- We need to learn ways to deal with unsafe situations and to make plans to avoid or deal with risk.
- We should be able to identify common health concerns in the community and to find ways to deal with those concerns.
- Changes in the size of families and the community affects the need for health services and community facilities. A bigger population needs more services.
- Drugs can have a short-term and a long-term effect on the health of people in the community.
- In some communities support is provided by different groups to help people deal with drugs.

Growth and development

BEHAVIOUR THAT HELPS US TO GROW AND DEVELOP

Everybody comes from a mother and a father and we usually look like our parents, although there will be some differences as well. Physical features or characteristics that we get from our parents are:

- colour of skin
- type of hair
- height
- shape of body
- facial features like the size and shape of nose

Because these characteristics are **inherited** from our parents, there is really nothing that we can do to change them. As we grow up we learn to accept the things that we cannot change.

We also know that there are things that we can change in our behaviour that will affect our growth and development. For example, we know that eating good food, taking regular exercise and having enough rest all help us to grow well. If our parents are tall then we may be able to grow tall too, but we will not grow tall unless we eat good food and get enough rest.

Behaviour that helps us to grow and develop includes the following:

- eating a balanced diet
- keeping fit and having exercise
- having enough rest and taking part in leisure activities
- keeping your brain active by exercises such as reading
- keeping clean and being hygienic—both your body and the surroundings
- living in a loving and caring environment
- having the support of family, friends and the community

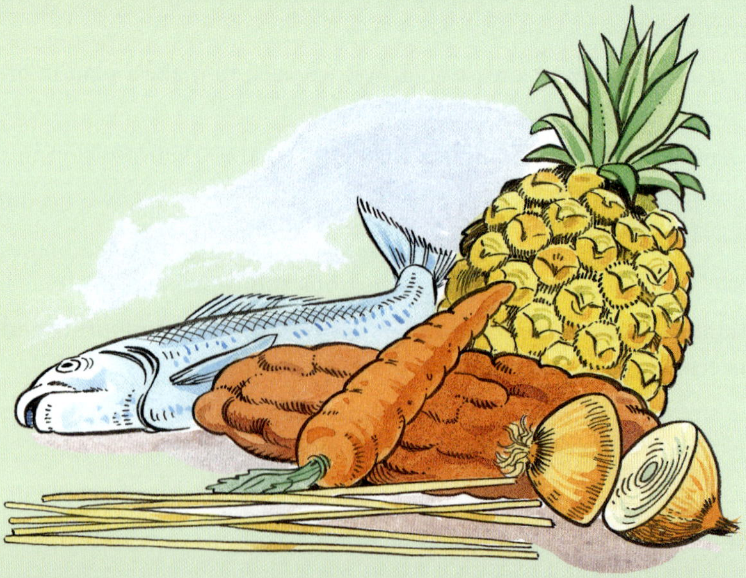

There are some conditions that come from the **environment** or influences from other people that may have a negative effect on our growth and development. For example:

- insects like mosquitoes that carry malaria
- pollution—breathing dirty or smoky air, drinking or washing in dirty water
- peer pressure—doing things because your friends do them, or because they 'force' you to do them

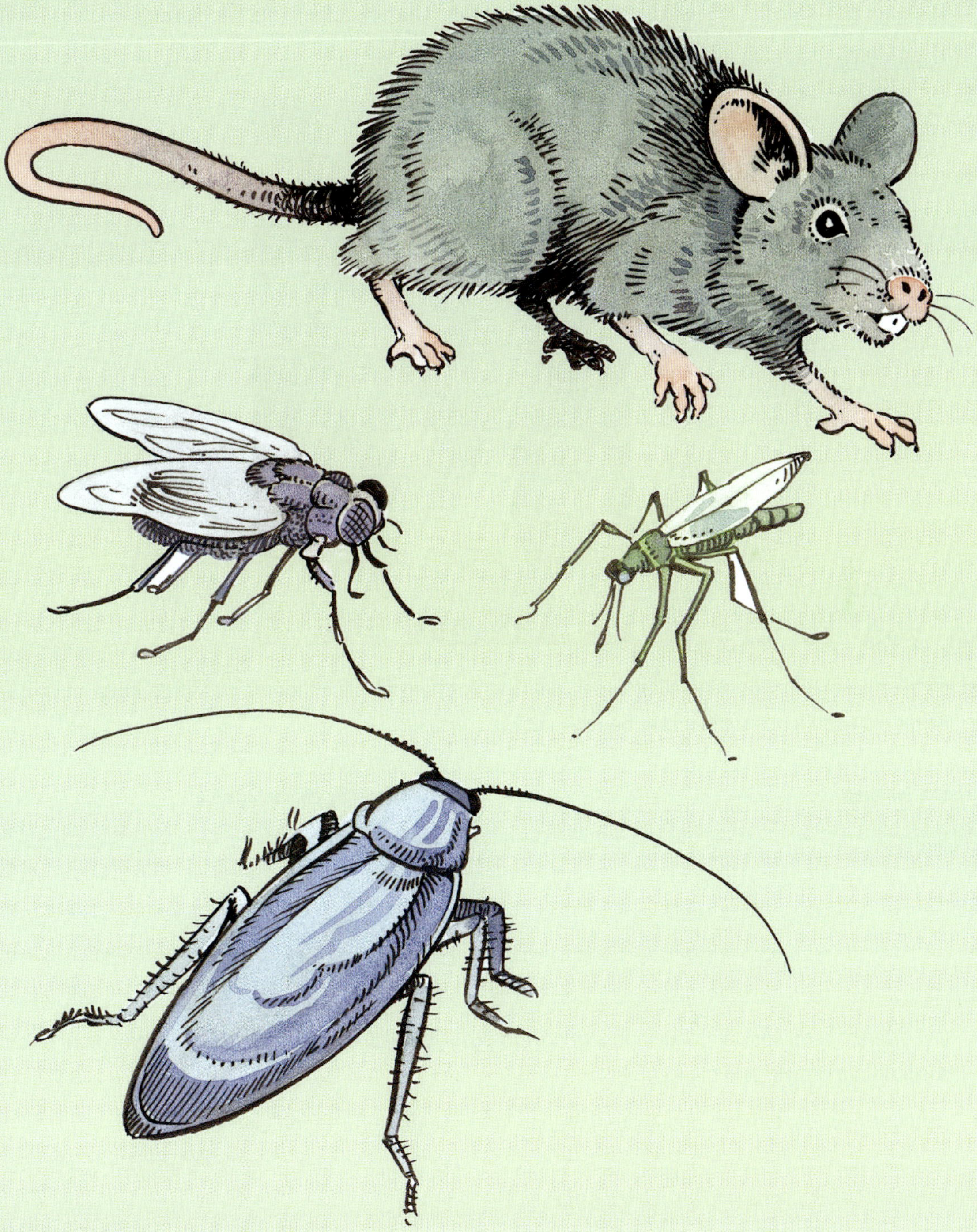

Responsibilities of parents

Being a parent is an important responsibility, and there are many things that parents need to do:

- take good care of the baby when the mother is pregnant by eating properly and by not smoking or drinking, both of which can harm the baby
- provide a balanced diet for children as far as possible
- teach children how to be good and useful members of the community
- decide to not smoke or use drugs and make sure that children do the same
- if they drink, then drink only a little and do not get drunk

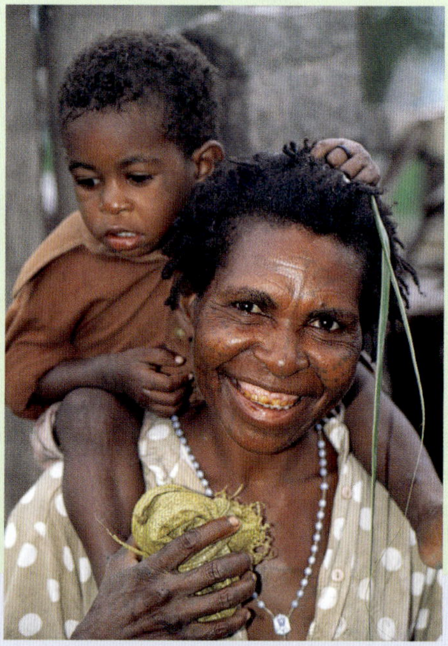

For you to try

- Make a list of your physical features and personality characteristics that are similar to those of your mother and father. You could use a table like the one below:

Physical features	Personality characteristics
Shape of nose	Sense of humour

- List different behaviour or conditions that have a positive effect on our growth and development or a negative effect on our growth and development.
- Describe how our families and cultural groups influence our growth and development.
- Describe the roles and responsibilities of parents and how they help their children to grow and develop properly.

WE ARE ALL DIFFERENT

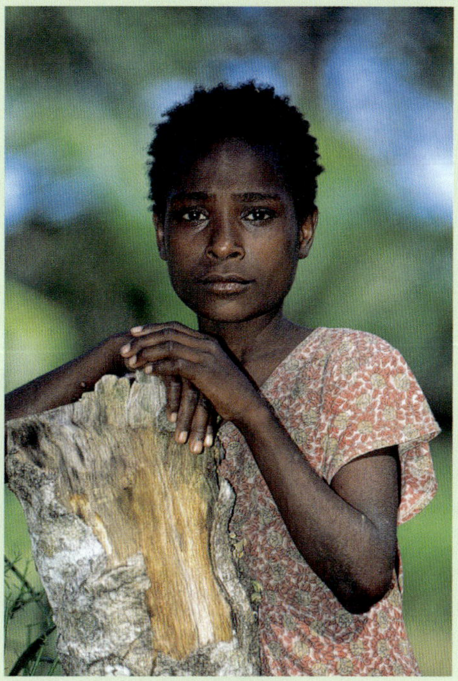

As you grow up, your body changes and you become sexually mature. This means that you are able to reproduce or have children. The stage in life when you develop from a child into an adult is called **puberty**. Girls usually start to grow up before boys, but everyone is different and it happens to everyone sooner or later, so we don't need to worry about what is normal.

The time between puberty and being a mature adult is known as adolescence. During adolescence you learn to think and behave as an adult. Adolescence can last for ten years or more and can be a difficult time for some young people, their parents and teachers. During this time you may find that your feelings are mixed up and your moods change quickly. For example, you may have strong feelings about such things as your family, your friends, your body or different kinds of music.

Some adolescents may feel shy or embarrassed or uncomfortable about themselves. In adolescence your body and feelings are changing, and it can sometimes take several years before you begin to know and accept yourself and have confidence to give your point of view or to make important decisions.

Another important development in adolescence is that girls begin to become more interested in boys and boys begin to become more interested in girls. These feelings of attraction can be very strong and are usually based on physical appearance. A boy may have strong feelings for a girl and she might not know or might not be interested, and it can also happen the other way around. Or a boy and a girl may feel love for each other but not have the maturity to know how to behave, or may not be allowed to meet because of the rules of the community.

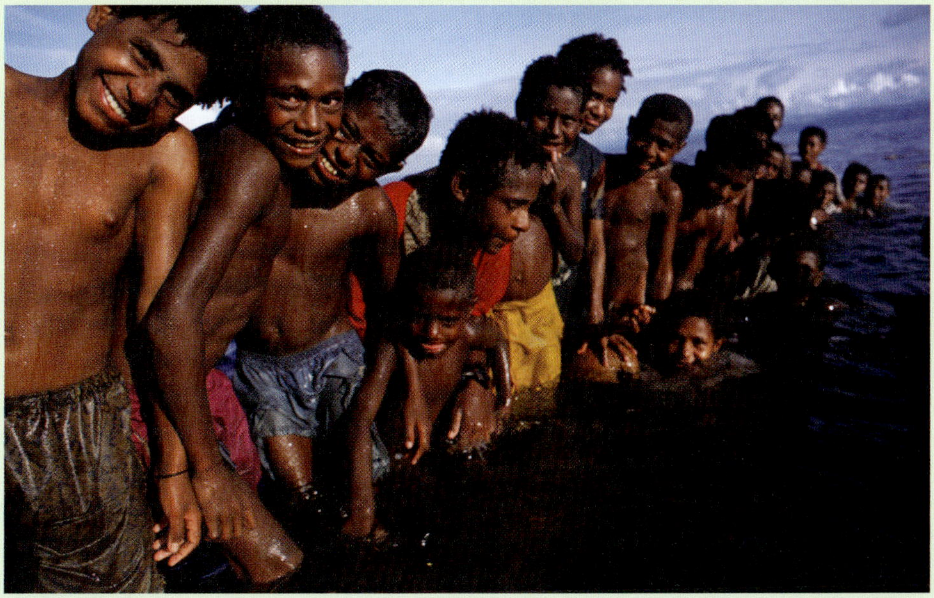

How individuals cope with changes

When you are having problems it often helps if you can talk with someone who understands. For example, you might talk to your friends or your parents, or to some other person in the community like an aunt or an uncle. Even if you are not having problems, it is still good to talk to others about what you are thinking and feeling.

The changes that take place during adolescence are part of your changing role in the community and show that you will soon be a part of adult society and will be able to take part in all the affairs of the community.

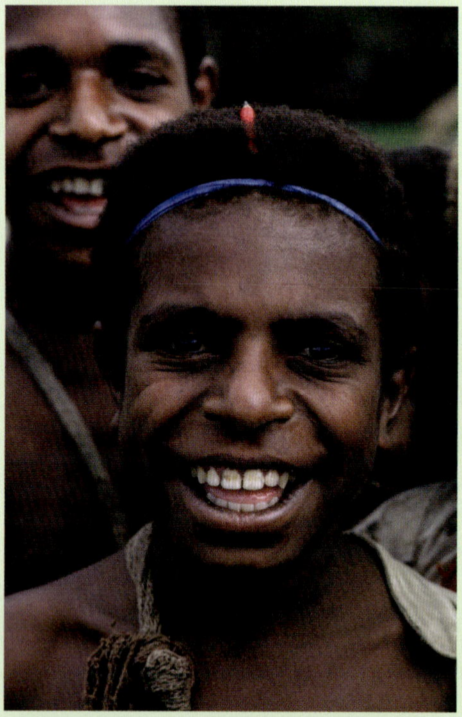

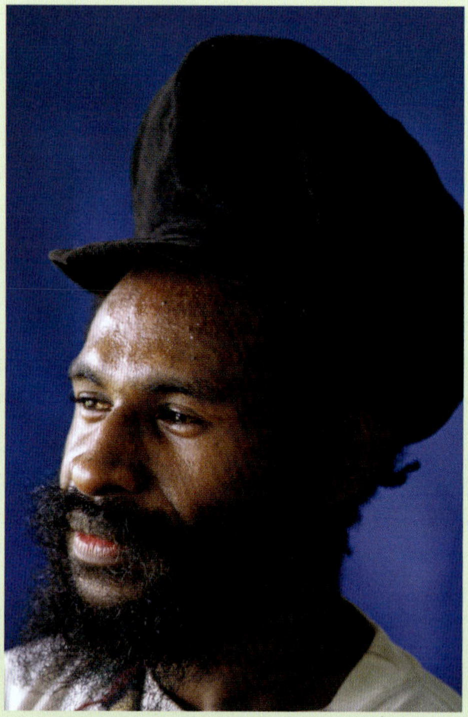

For you to try

- Draw a series of circles that are linked like the ones below. Write some issues concerning adolescence in each circle. Write words that show your feelings about each issue. One example has been completed for you.

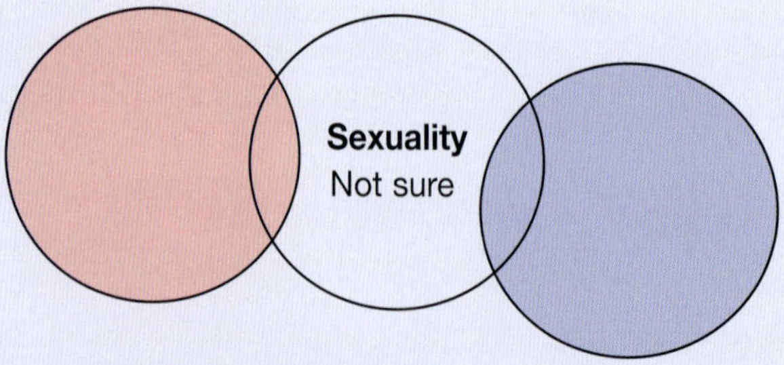

- Use the decision-making model that you learned in 'Living and Working Together' in Grade 6 to discuss with a partner what you would do to sort out different problems or issues.

CULTURAL BELIEFS AND VALUES ABOUT SEXUALITY (M)

As well as the physical changes that take place during puberty, there are also social and emotional changes. You develop a sense of your own sexuality—the way that you think and feel and behave as a young man or young woman. You develop values, beliefs and behaviour that may be influenced by traditional ideas about what it means to be a man or a woman.

You will probably become interested in new types of relationships, like having a boyfriend or girlfriend. You will begin to have choices and make decisions about your sexual behaviour.

During puberty and adolescence, the following are likely to be important to young people:

- The changes that take place during puberty may make some people worried or feel shame.
- You will begin to have sexual thoughts and feelings. It is normal and healthy to have these, although many people do not feel comfortable talking about them. We have to learn how to behave as a result of the thoughts and feelings that we have.
- Your relations with others of the same sex and the opposite sex will change and are likely to become more important.
- You will have questions about sexual behaviour like sexual intercourse. What is it like? When is the right time to have sexual intercourse?

Our feelings and understanding of sexuality are likely to be influenced by the following:

- being male or female—boys and girls often see the same thing in a different way
- family beliefs and values
- culture
- religion
- peers
- our emotional and physical feelings at different times
- the media—newspapers and magazines, radio and television, films.

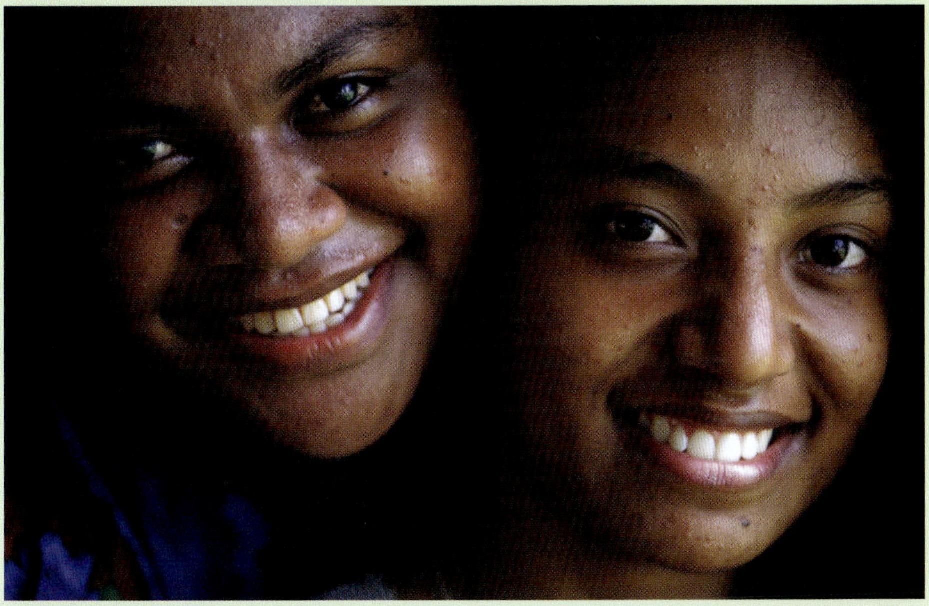

ATTITUDES TO SEXUALITY

One of the most important attitudes to sexuality is **equality**. This means that girls have the same rights as boys and women have the same rights as men. Boys should not try to make girls behave in certain ways just because they are stronger. Girls often see sexual matters in a different way from boys, and we should always respect the point of view of each person. One person should never force another to do something that they do not want to do.

People from different cultural groups often have different beliefs about what is appropriate behaviour or what are appropriate ways to express sexuality. For example, in some cultures it is acceptable for boys and girls to meet together at night, but in other cultures this is not allowed. In the Highlands, groups of boys and girls sometimes meet inside the house for a ceremony called 'turnim head' in which a boy sits opposite a girl with their faces close together and turn their heads so that their lips and noses rub together. In the Trobriand Islands of Milne Bay a boy and a girl can meet at night, but this is done carefully so that no one knows about it.

Another important attitude that we need in our sexual behaviour is **responsibility**. Sexual feelings are often very strong, but just because your body is physically ready to have a sexual relationship does not mean that you are emotionally mature and ready to cope with the results. You need to think carefully before having or starting a sexual relationship.

For example, having sexual intercourse can lead to pregnancy or **sexually transmitted infections** or even HIV/AIDS. Having a baby that you do not want can also cause a lot of worry, especially for the girl, who may try to hide the fact that she is pregnant for as long as possible. It is better to wait until you know that you are both ready to bring up a baby, and to know how to prevent pregnancy and sexually transmitted infections, before you start to have sexual intercourse.

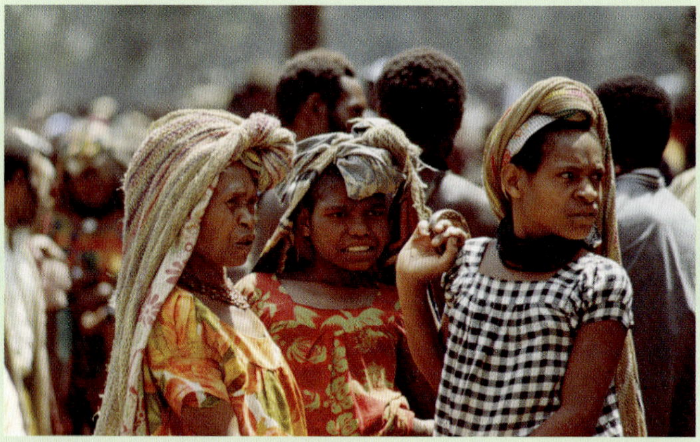

Women have the same rights as men

For you to try

- Discuss with a partner when is the right time to have a sexual relationship.
- List the things that you need to consider before you start a sexual relationship.
- A Imagine that someone is trying to force you to have a sexual relationship or to do something that you do not want to do. What can you do to cope with this pressure? Write down the things that you would say as well as the things that you would do.

Nutrition

REASONS FOR PEOPLE'S FOOD CHOICES ML

The type of food that we eat and the way that it is cooked is one of the most important differences between people from different countries and from different provinces or regions of a country. When we visit another place or go and live in another place, one of the first things that we notice is the food. If we cannot get the food that we like, then we may feel unsatisfied.

Sometimes people arrange for food to be sent from their home to the place where they are living. For example, village people in Papua New Guinea often send baskets of food to their relatives or students who are living in town. In the same way, people from Western Samoa send food to their relatives who are living in New Zealand. Taro does not grow in New Zealand, so relatives often send big boxes of taro by airfreight. Taro is the **staple food** of people from Western Samoa and they like to eat this food every day, even if they are living a long way from home.

Some reasons for the choice of food are:

- what can be easily grown in the area
- the time and effort needed to prepare the food
- the nutritional value of the food—will it be good for us?
- the availability of food—what food is in the market or the store?
- the cost of food—what can people afford to buy?
- cultural and religious beliefs, practices and taboos that allow people to eat some foods but not others—what foods are we allowed to eat?

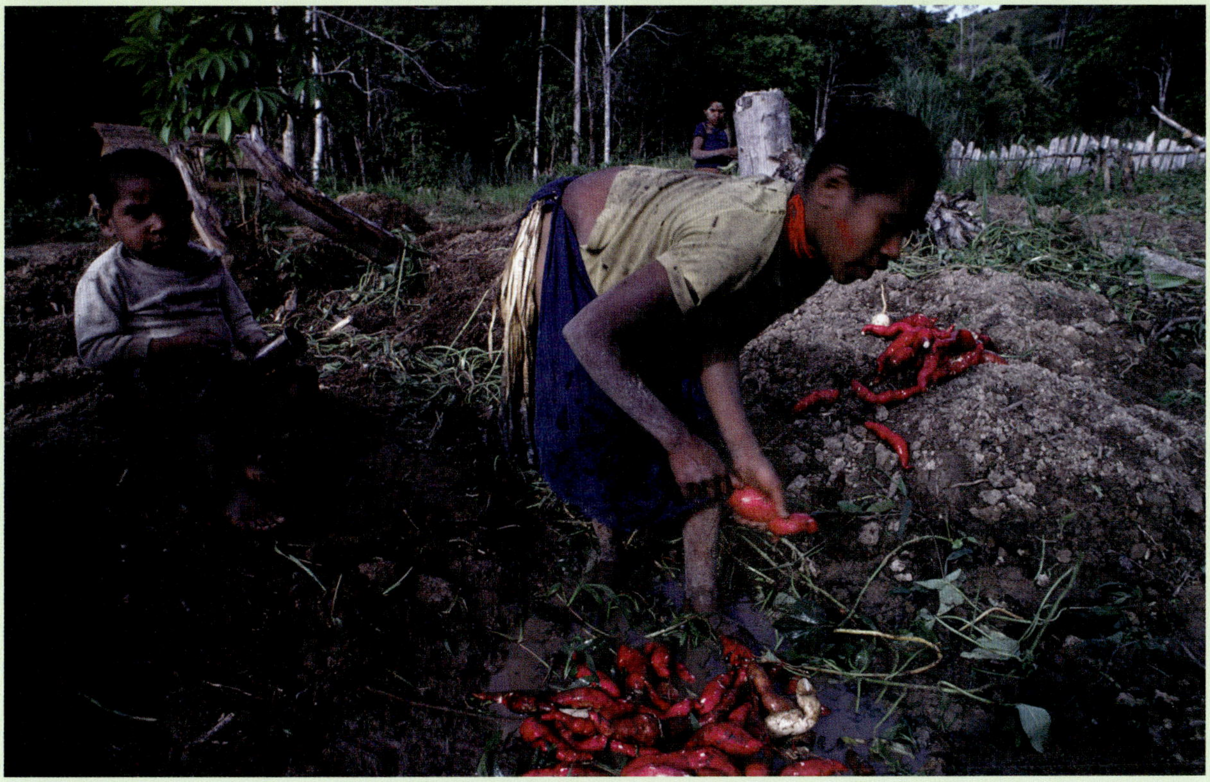

The food choices that people make may also be influenced or affected by the following:

- their personal preferences for different types of food
- the need to eat some foods because a woman is pregnant or because a young person is still growing
- the type of lifestyle that a person is living—people who are very busy may not have enough time to cook some foods or to use some cooking methods
- a health problem that means people may need to eat more or less of a particular kind of food. For example, people with **diabetes** need to be careful about the amount of sugar in their diet. People with **anaemia**, especially girls and women, who do not have enough iron in their blood, need to eat plenty of dark green leafy vegetables like aibika.
- cultural background—some cultures encourage or discourage certain types of food. For example, some people do not like to eat pork.
- family size—the amount and type of food may be limited in a large family
- advertising, which may encourage people to eat certain types of take-away food or fast food, especially in urban areas.

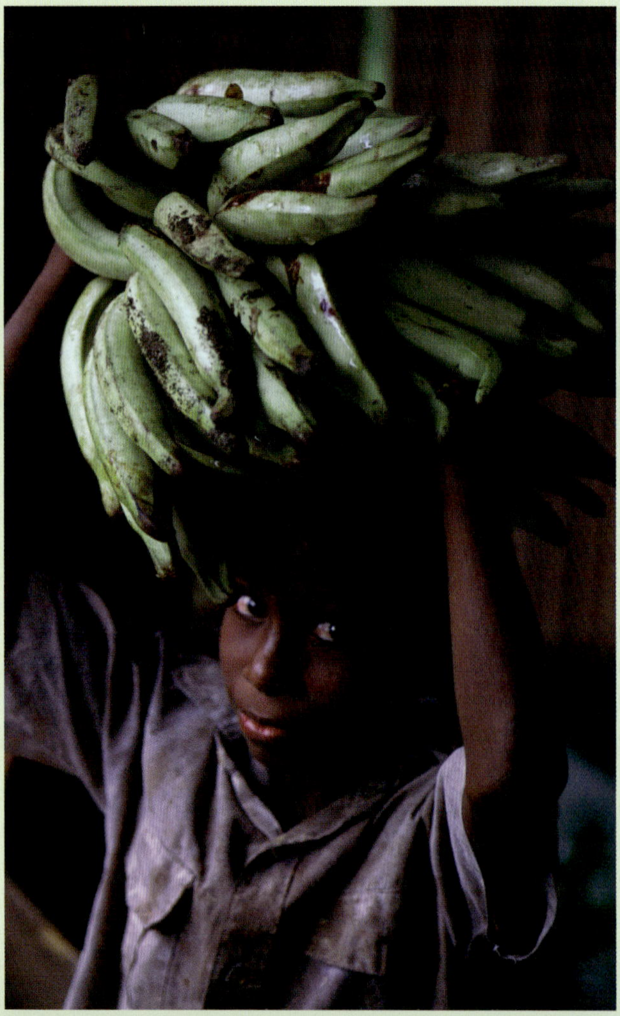

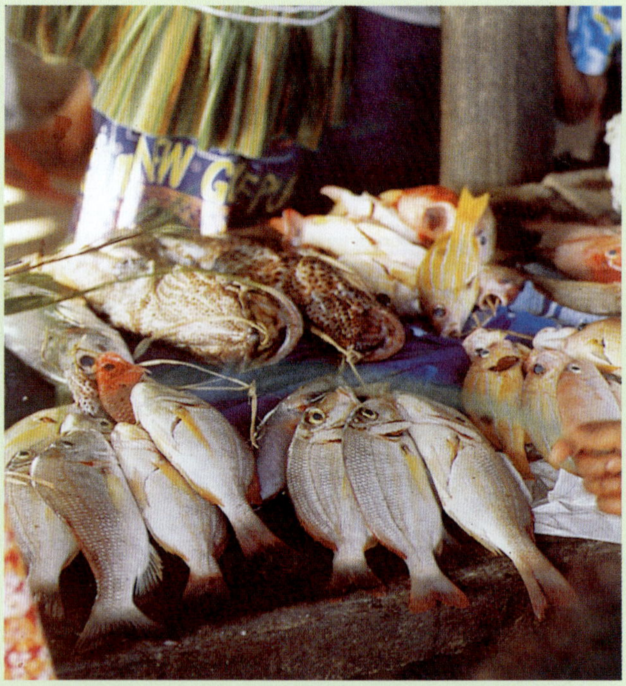

For you to try

- List some of the major influences on people's food choices.
- Describe the foods that are prepared and eaten by your cultural group or a group that you know well.
- Find out about some beliefs or myths associated with particular kinds of food and the way that they are prepared. Write about one of these myths or beliefs.
- Carry out a survey in your school or community to find out about people who need a special diet or who have special nutritional needs. What are the influences on their diet? How can the food that they eat be checked or monitored?

NUTRITION IN YOUR SCHOOL AND COMMUNITY ML

When we eat, it is important to eat food that will help to make us healthy. Food contains substances called **nutrients**. The purpose of nutrients and the foods in which they are found are shown in the table below:

Purpose of the nutrient	Where is the nutrient found?
Supply energy to the body	Carbohydrates (sugar and starchy foods) and fat
Normal growth, development and repair of damaged parts of the body	Protein is needed for growth, and vitamins found in fresh fruit and vegetables can help with healing
Normal functioning and regulation of the body	Minerals found in different foods and fibre found in many vegetables
Resistance to disease and infection	Vitamins found in fresh fruit and vegetables

When we eat enough of the right kinds of food then we are eating a **balanced diet**. People who do not eat a balanced diet are more likely to become sick. For example, if we do not eat enough fresh fruit and vegetables, then we do not have enough vitamins in our diet to protect against disease and infection.

If we do not have enough protein in our diet then we will not grow properly, and when we injure ourselves our body will be slow to repair itself. For example, if you cut yourself or have a bad sore then your body will heal the wound, but if your diet is low in protein and vitamins then the wound will heal very slowly.

We need enough carbohydrate food (such as sweet potato, rice and sugar) to provide energy to do work. If we do not eat enough carbohydrate, then we will not be able to do physical activity like working in the garden, walking or playing sport. When we eat more carbohydrate than we need we become overweight, which is not healthy.

We need fat in our diet to help keep us warm, to protect organs and to provide energy. However, when we eat too much fat we can become overweight and it can become hard for the blood to be pumped around the body. Eating a diet that contains a lot of fat can lead to health problems, especially when the person does not do enough exercise and also smokes cigarettes.

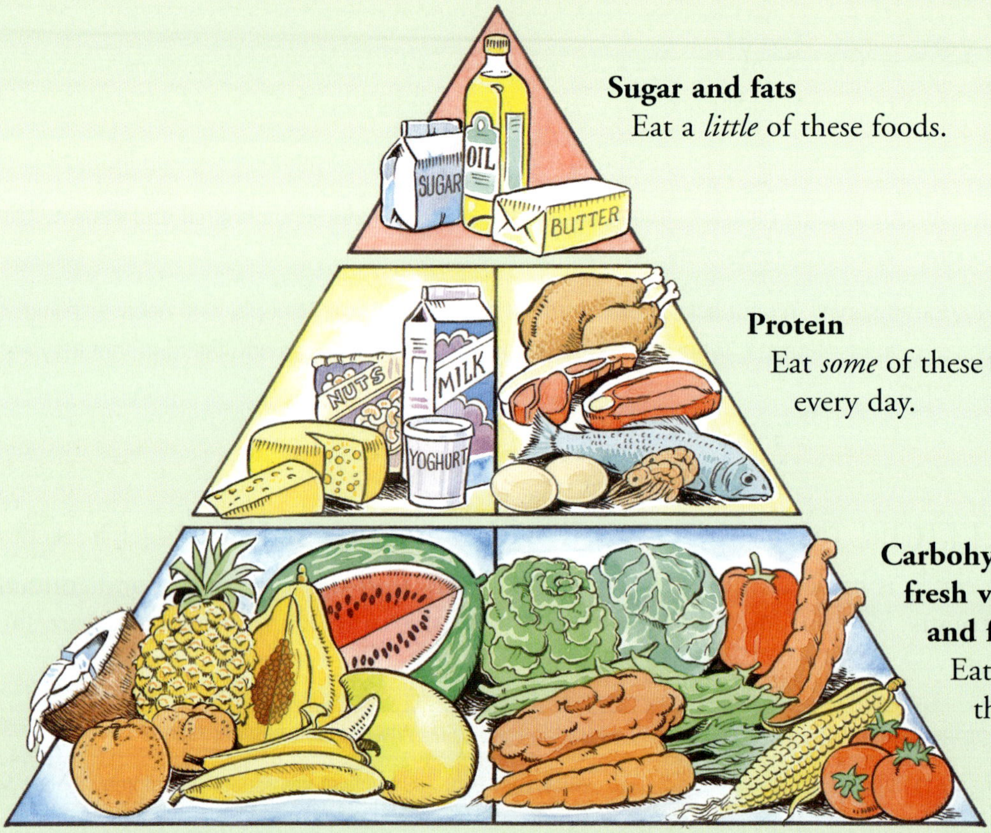

Sugar and fats
Eat a *little* of these foods.

Protein
Eat *some* of these foods every day.

Carbohydrates, fresh vegetables and fruits
Eat *most* of these foods.

NUTRITION CHECKLIST (ML)

Everybody in the community should eat a balanced diet, but the diet of young people is even more important. Children who do not get enough of the right kinds of food will not grow and develop well and will not be able to learn properly in school. This means that we should eat nutritious food at home and outside the home.

We can find out whether we are eating a balanced diet by using a nutrition checklist to record the food that we ate for a whole week. It is important to include all the food that is eaten, including any snack food and food that is eaten outside the home. We need to record the nutrients that are found in the food and also make a comment to say if there was too much or not enough of a particular type of food. An example for one day is shown in the table:

Name: Lani	**Date: Week beginning October 25**		
Day/meal	**Food eaten**	**Nutrients**	**Comment for the day or week—too much or not enough?**
Monday breakfast	Hard biscuit, tea with sugar	Carbohydrate (starch and sugar)	No fruit
Monday lunch	Sweet potato, corn, peanuts	Carbohydrate, protein	
Monday dinner	Rice, fish, aibika	Carbohydrate, protein, fat, vitamins, minerals	

We need to look at the food that is eaten for a whole week, not just one day. In the example, Lani did not eat any fruit on Monday. This does not matter too much, but if she did not eat any fruit for a long period of time, then she may not be getting enough vitamins.

Because food that is eaten outside the home is important, we need to think about the food that we buy at school or snack foods that we buy at the store. Many takeaway or fast foods are fried and so contain a lot of fat or added salt or sugar. Eating too much of these fast foods is not healthy. Schools should not sell unhealthy foods in the canteen or tuck shop, and when we sell food on special occasions like a school celebration, we should prepare healthy food.

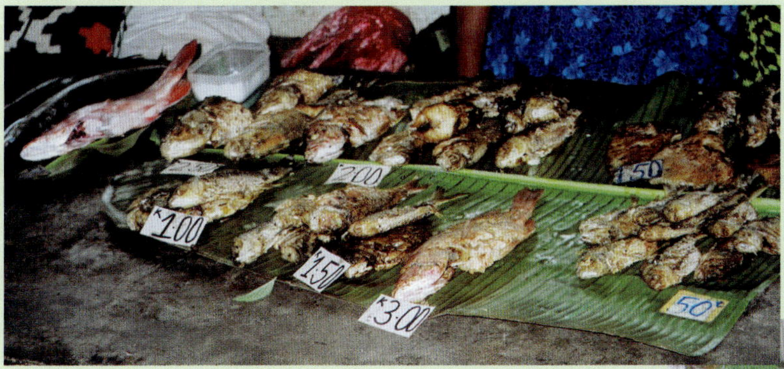

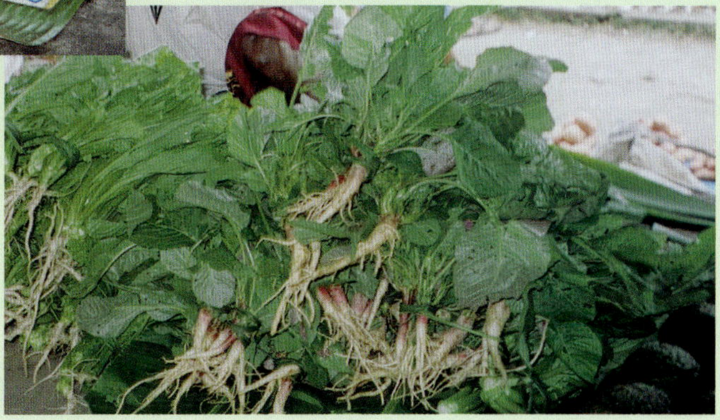

For you to try

- What do students in your school eat for lunch? Do they bring their own food or buy food at school? Carry out a survey to answer these questions.
- Does your school have rules or a policy about school lunch—especially the things that can be sold to students? If not, work out some rules or guidelines about lunch in your school. If your school already has a school lunch policy then say how these rules can be improved.
- What type of food is eaten by the people in your community? How does the food they eat affect the health of the people?
- Think about a situation in which young people are not eating a healthy diet, like eating too many sweet foods or fried food. Suggest a way or a strategy that could be used to get them to change their diet.
- How can the type of food that is available in your school be improved? Prepare a report and make recommendations to start a school canteen.

Personal health and safety

HEALTH ISSUES THAT ARE IMPORTANT TO YOUNG PEOPLE ML

When you are young you are still learning about many different things and learning to make your own decisions. We all want to feel that we belong to a group and when you are young this feeling can be very strong. This means that you may find you are doing things because other young people are doing those things. They may even try to force you to do certain things. This is called **peer pressure**.

You need to think for yourself and make your own decisions to make sure that you do the things that will keep you healthy, even if your friends are doing something that is not healthy. You should not do something just because your friends are doing it, and you should not do something if your friends force you to do it. It can be quite hard to behave in ways that are different from your friends, but in the end people will respect you more for making up your own mind and staying with your decision.

For example, young people have to decide what they will do about the following:

- using drugs such as smoking cigarettes or using other illegal substances like marijuana
- drinking alcohol
- chewing betel nut
- taking exercise
- body image
- grooming and dressing
- the type of food eaten, such as sweets and greasy food
- sexual activity that can lead to sexually transmitted infections, including HIV

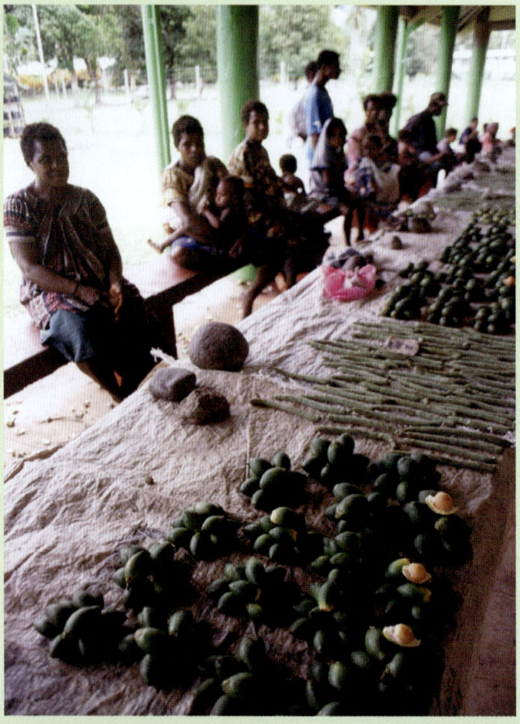

Selling betel nut at a market

HEALTH GOALS

One good way to help you to make good choices is to have **health goals**. These are the things that you will aim for because they will help to keep you safe and healthy. For example:

- Take regular exercise—at least three or four times per week.
- Develop good personal hygiene—wash your body and hair regularly and brush your teeth. Change your clothes when they need changing.
- Develop positive relationships with other people.
- Develop positive self-esteem so that you feel good about yourself.
- Be assertive when you need to be so you can clearly state your point of view.
- Learn to say 'no' to the things that you do not want to do, for example, taking drugs and having sex.
- Avoid situations that are unsafe or threatening.
- Learn how to cope with different situations, including those that are difficult.

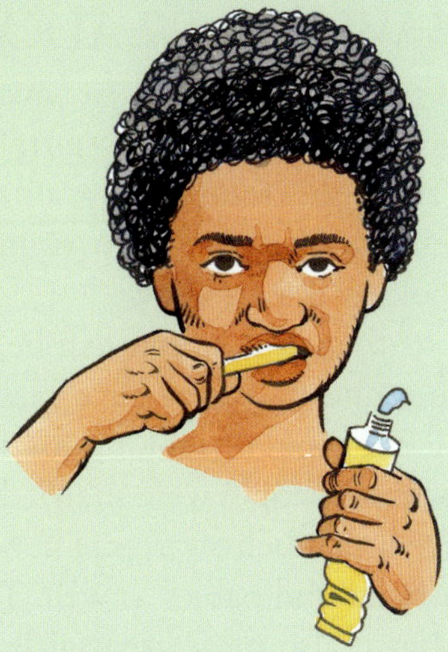

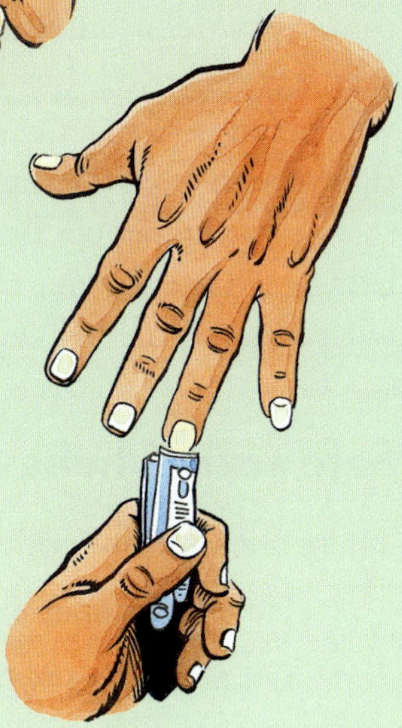

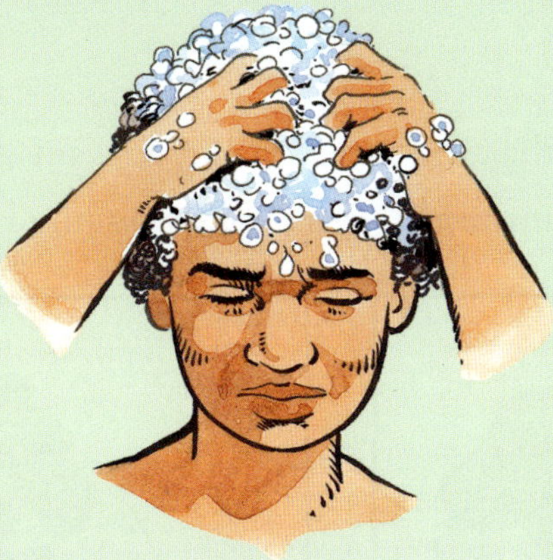

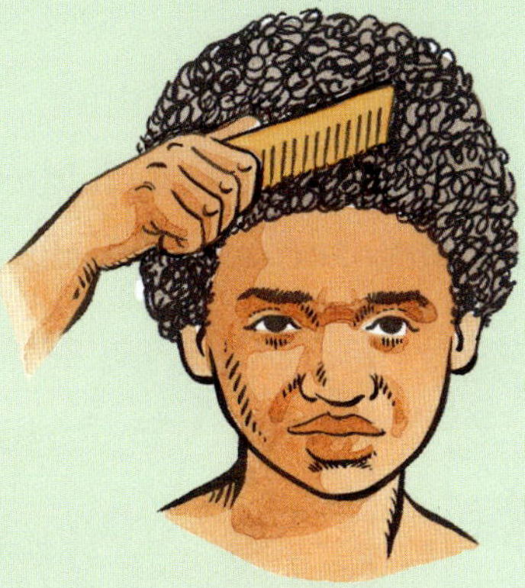

For you to try

- Make a list of the health issues that are most important to you and your friends. Describe how these issues can affect you.
- How do your friends or other people in your community handle or solve different health problems? Carry out a survey to find out about the ways that they do this.
- What people or groups are there in your community who can help young people with their health problems? How do you get the information that you need from these people?

SEXUAL BEHAVIOUR IN ADOLESCENCE

When a girl reaches puberty and starts to have her periods it means that she can become a mother, and when a boy reaches puberty and he starts to produce sperm it means that he can become a father. Girls and boys also develop strong feelings of attraction for one another and feel like having sexual intercourse, but during adolescence most young people are not ready to cope with looking after a wife or a husband and looking after a baby.

One of the reasons that adolescence can be a difficult time for young people is because their bodies are ready to reproduce and they may have these strong feelings to have sexual intercourse. However, because they are still in school or looking for a job, they are not ready to start a family as well. In many traditional societies people were married soon after they became reached puberty so that the period of adolescence was much shorter. They then had to make their own gardens and learn to take care of a wife or husband and babies as well. This helped to prevent young people having babies before they were married, but it also meant that girls had their first baby when they were still teenagers, which can be dangerous for the girl. Pregnancy is a dangerous time for all women, but especially when the woman is very young.

For young people in many countries, including Papua New Guinea, the time between puberty and being ready to get married and start a family can be ten years or more. So young people have to decide what their sexual behaviour will be in this time.

Safe sexual behaviour

There are a number of things that you can do in order to stay safe:

- Have only one sexual partner.
- Do not have sex outside marriage—be faithful.
- Use contraception to have the number of children that you want, when you want them.
- Use condoms to prevent pregnancy and sexually transmitted infections, including HIV.

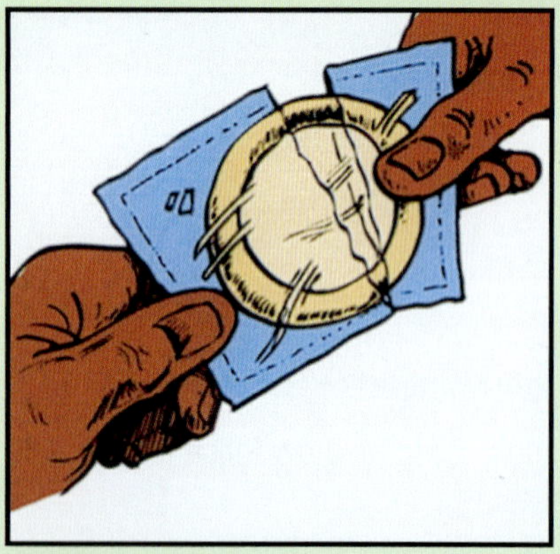

Carefully remove the condom from the packet. Be careful not to tear the condom. Make sure it is the right way round so it can be unrolled.

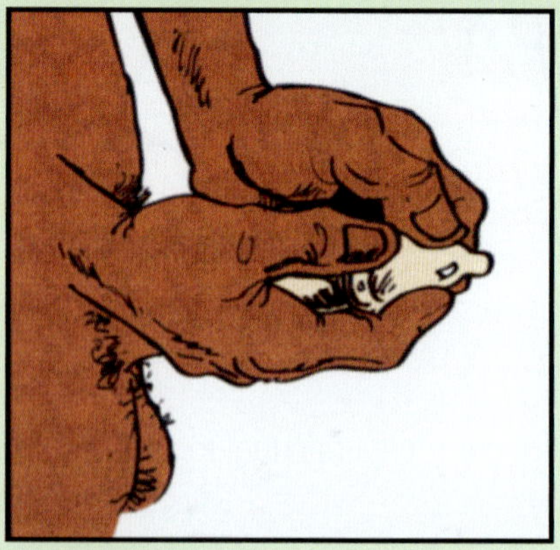

Put the condom on once the penis is hard. Squeeze the air out of the tip of the condom first.

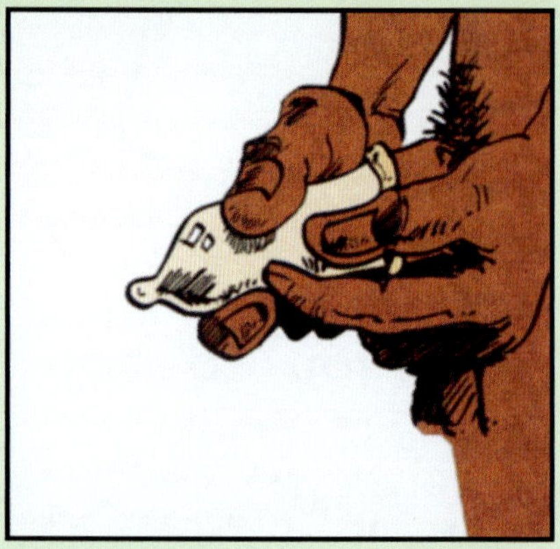

Unroll the condom all the way along the penis.

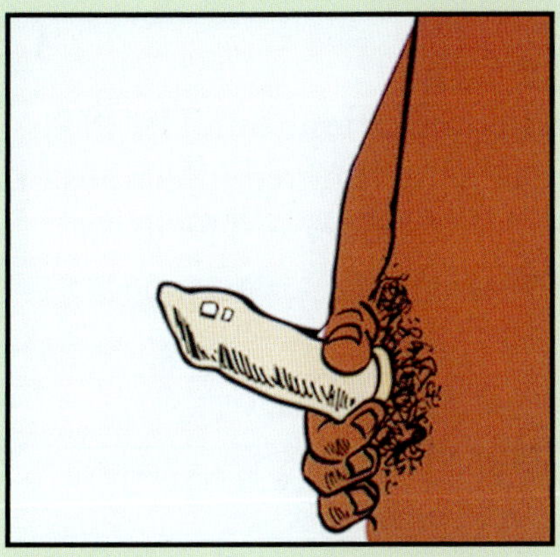

Make sure there is no air in the end of the condom.

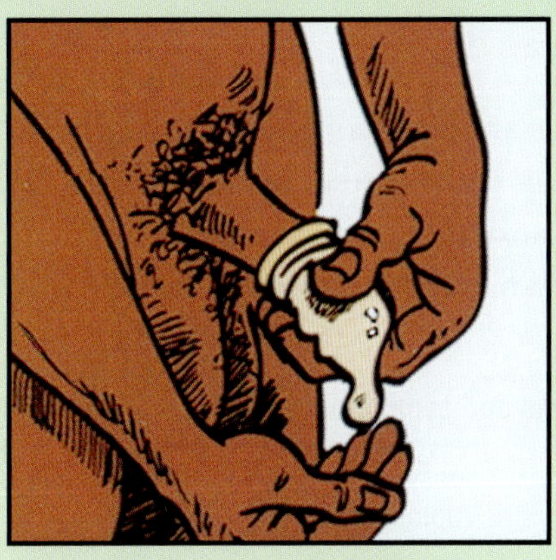

Soon after sex, take the penis out holding onto the condom. Tie the open end of the condom in a knot and put it in a rubbish bin.

Sexual responsibilities

Every person has responsibilities in their sexual behaviour to do the following:

- Respect yourself and others.
- Stay faithful to your partner.
- Use condoms to prevent pregnancy and sexually transmitted infections.

Values that influence our behaviour and decision-making

The way that we behave is influenced by the values that we have—by all the things that we think or say are important. For example:

- personal integrity—being truthful and honest to yourself and others
- respect for the dignity of other people
- respect for the values of other people
- respect for the values of the community
- obligations to your family and the community
- being caring—ready and able to look after others
- being compassionate—being kind and understanding what someone else is feeling
- being dependable—so that someone else can rely on you
- being tolerant—so that you do not get angry easily
- being considerate—so that you can think of other people
- being cooperative—so that you can work with others
- being willing to accept responsibility and share in decision-making

Unsafe sexual behaviour

The risks of unsafe sexual behaviour are pregnancy and **sexually transmitted infections** or STIs. (STIs are also sometimes known as sexually transmitted diseases or STDs.) Sexually transmitted infections or STIs can only be caught by having sexual intercourse with someone who has the disease. The main STIs in Papua New Guinea are shown in the following table:

STI	Cause	Signs and symptoms	Treatment
Gonorrhoea	bacteria	Pain on passing urine. A discharge of pus from the penis or vagina.	Injection with the antibiotic penicillin
Syphilis	bacteria	Painless sores on the penis or vagina with hard, raised edges which give out a colourless liquid.	Injection with the antibiotic penicillin
Donovanosis	bacteria	Ulcers which eat away the penis or vagina.	Injection with the antibiotic chloramphenicol
HIV/AIDS	virus	Weakens the body's immune system so that there is no protection to infection from disease. For example, people may have pneumonia, tuberculosis, brain infections and very bad diarrhoea.	Very little treatment in PNG. Cannot be cured. Most people with AIDS die.

Most STIs can be treated with antibiotics, so if you think that you might have caught a sexually transmitted infection then you should go and get treatment as soon as possible. Many people feel shame about going to get treatment, but it is important to overcome this feeling. The nurses and doctors are trained to deal with this problem in a way that does not make the patient feel ashamed. Some STIs like gonorrhoea appear to get better by themselves, but they can come back later on and the person can die.

HIV/AIDS is becoming a big problem in Papua New Guinea. Unfortunately, there is no cure and most of the people who get HIV will die.

If you do not have sexual intercourse before you get married, and then if both husband and wife have sex only with each other, you will not catch a sexually transmitted infection.

For you to try

- How will you protect yourself against pressures to have sexual intercourse before you are ready? Write a list of things that you will do and say if someone tries to force you to do something.
- Make groups of four or five students. Discuss different age groups and identify the high risk groups for different kinds of sexual behaviour.
- In a role play, show some things that you can do to prevent unsafe sexual behaviour in different situations.
- List the symptoms of different STIs.

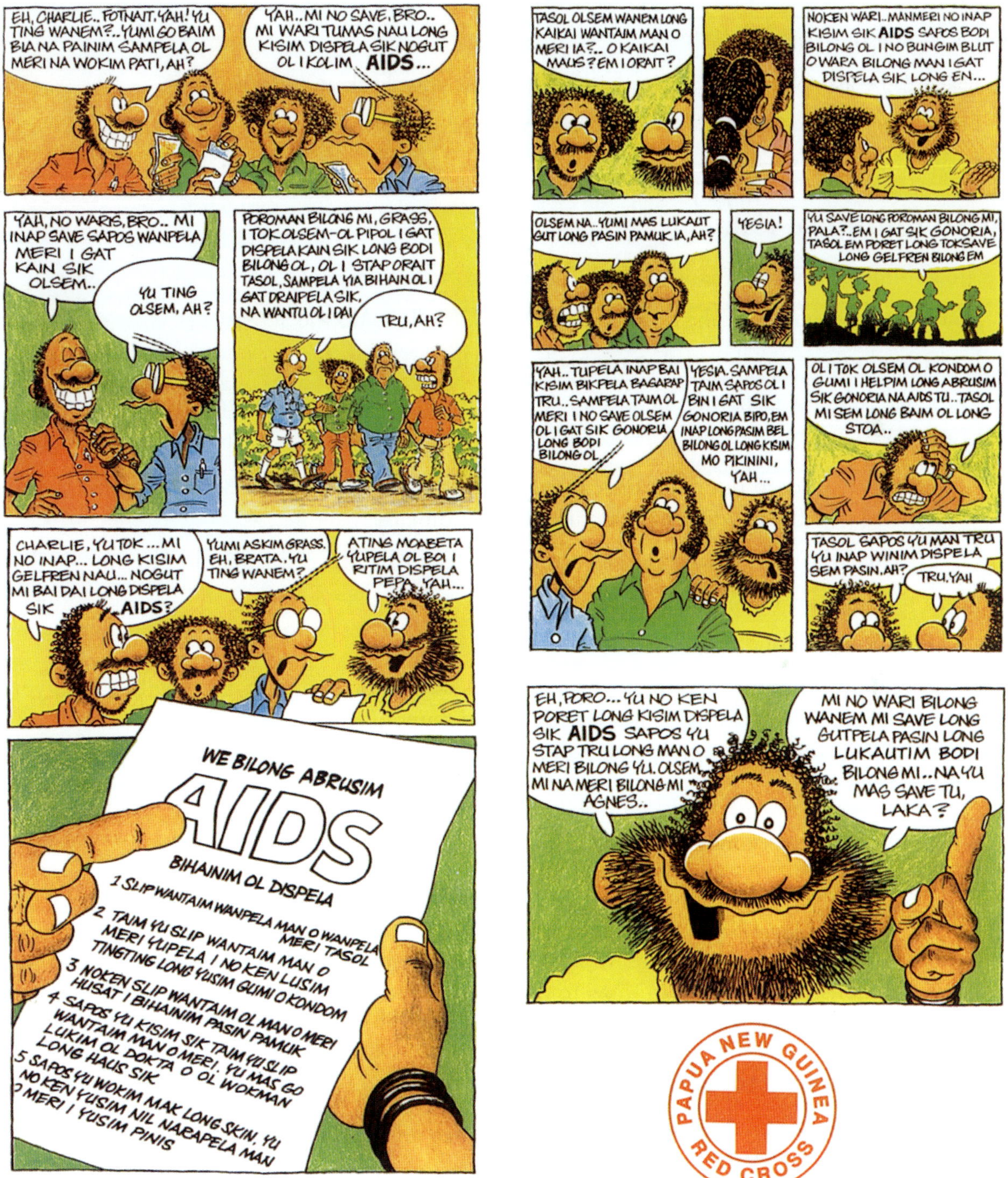
EH, CHARLIE.. FOTNAIT, YAH! YU TING WANEM?.. YUMI GO BAIM BIA NA PAINIM SAMPELA OL MERI NA WOKIM PATI, AH?
YAH.. MI NO SAVE, BRO.. MI WARI TUMAS NAU LONG KISIM DISPELA SIK NOGUT OL I KOLIM AIDS...
YAH, NO WARIS, BRO.. MI INAP SAVE SAPOS WANPELA MERI I GAT KAIN SIK OLSEM..
YU TING OLSEM, AH?
POROMAN BILONG MI, GRASS, I TOK OLSEM—OL PIPOL I GAT DISPELA KAIN SIK LONG BODI BILONG OL, OL I STAP ORAIT TASOL, SAMPELA YIA BIHAIN OL I GAT DRAIPELA SIK, NA WANTU OL I DAI
TRU, AH?
CHARLIE, YU TOK... MI NO INAP... LONG KISIM GELFREN NAU... NOGUT MI BAI DAI LONG DISPELA SIK AIDS?
YUMI ASKIM GRASS. EH, BRATA, YU TING WANEM?
ATING MOABETA YUPELA OL BOI I RITIM DISPELA PEPA, YAH...
WE BILONG ABRUSIM
AIDS
BIHAINIM OL DISPELA
1 SLIP WANTAIM WANPELA MAN O WANPELA MERI TASOL
2 TAIM YU SLIP WANTAIM MAN O MERI YUPELA I NO KEN LUSIM TINGTING LONG YUSIM GUMI O KONDOM
3 NOKEN SLIP WANTAIM OL MAN O MERI HUSAT I BIHAINIM PASIN PAMUK
4 SAPOS YU KISIM SIK TAIM YU SLIP WANTAIM MAN O MERI, YU MAS GO LUKIM OL DOKTA O OL WOKMAN LONG HAUS SIK
5 SAPOS YU WOKIM MAK LONG SKIN, YU NO KEN YUSIM NIL NARAPELA MAN O MERI I YUSIM PINIS
TASOL OLSEM WANEM LONG KAIKAI WANTAIM MAN O MERI IA?.. O KAIKAI MAUS? EM I ORAIT?
NOKEN WARI.. MANMERI NO INAP KISIM SIK AIDS SAPOS BODI BILONG OL I NO BUNGIM BLUT O WARA BILONG MAN I GAT DISPELA SIK LONG EN...
OLSEM NA.. YUMI MAS LUKAUT GUT LONG PASIN PAMUK IA, AH?
YESIA!
YU SAVE LONG POROMAN BILONG MI, PALA?.. EM I GAT SIK GONORIA, TASOL EM PORET LONG TOKSAVE LONG GELFREN BILONG EM
YAH.. TUPELA INAP BAI KISIM BIKPELA BAGARAP TRU.. SAMPELA TAIM OL MERI I NO SAVE OLSEM OL I GAT SIK GONORIA LONG BODI BILONG OL
YESIA. SAMPELA TAIM SAPOS OL I BIN I GAT SIK GONORIA BIPO, EM INAP LONG PASIM BEL BILONG OL LONG KISIM MO PIKININI, YAH...
OL I TOK OLSEM OL KONDOM O GUMI I HELPIM LONG ABRUSIM SIK GONORIA NA AIDS TU.. TASOL MI SEM LONG BAIM OL LONG STOA..
TASOL SAPOS YU MAN TRU YU INAP WINIM DISPELA SEM PASIN, AH?
TRU, YAH
EH, PORO... YU NO KEN PORET LONG KISIM DISPELA SIK AIDS SAPOS YU STAP TRU LONG MAN O MERI BILONG YU. OLSEM, MI NA MERI BILONG MI AGNES..
MI NO WARI BILONG WANEM MI SAVE LONG GUTPELA PASIN LONG LUKAUTIM BODI BILONG MI.. NA YU MAS SAVE TU, LAKA?

PAPUA NEW GUINEA RED CROSS

WAYS TO RESPOND TO UNSAFE SITUATIONS

Even though we take care and try to avoid danger, there will be times when we find ourselves in an unsafe situation. It helps if we know how to respond. Some ways to respond to unsafe situations are as follows:

- Learn to assess risks.
- Learn to be assertive—to be confident to say what you think about something.
- Learn how to protect yourself if someone threatens you or hits you.
- Learn how to do first-aid.

How to minimise risk

There are a number of things that we can do in order to reduce the risk of a particular activity:

- Make sure that you have the right equipment and skills to do the activity.
- Learn road safety and show other people how to follow the rules.
- Learn the rules for using fire. Learn how to use primus stoves and pressure lanterns safely.
- Learn how to put out a fire:
  - — Never use water to put out a fire caused by electricity—you can get an electric shock. Instead use sand or a fire extinguisher that uses carbon dioxide.
  - — A person who has burning clothes can be wrapped in a mat or blanket to put out the flames.
- Learn the rules for water safety.
  - — Do not swim alone.
  - — Do not dive unless you know that the water is deep enough and that you will not hit your head on a log or rock that is hidden under the water.
  - — Do not try to cross rivers that are flowing very fast.
  - — Do not travel on canoes or boats that are overloaded or not safe.
  - — Do not travel by canoe or boat when the weather is not good.
- Learn how to use tools properly and to store them safely—especially any tools that have a sharp cutting edge.
- If you use chemicals like pesticides to kill pests in the garden, read the label carefully and follow the instructions so that you learn how to use them properly. Learn the proper way to store chemicals.

Actions to respond to unsafe situations

There are a number of things that we can do to respond to an unsafe situation:

- Remove yourself from the situation. You may need to move very quickly when you are in danger, but make sure that you do not run into more danger.
- Tell other people about the danger so that they can avoid the situation.
- If possible, try to make the situation safer or to reduce the danger.

Actions to respond to emergency situations

There are a number of things that we can do to respond to an emergency situation:

- Keep calm and think clearly so that you can make a decision about the situation for yourself and other people.
- Remove yourself and other people from the danger.
- If there are rules about the situation then follow the rules. For example, in the case of a fire in a building, everyone should know how to leave the building and where to meet outside so that you know that everyone is safe.
- Get help when it is needed. You need to know where the nearest help is and who to ask.
- Give first aid to people who need it.

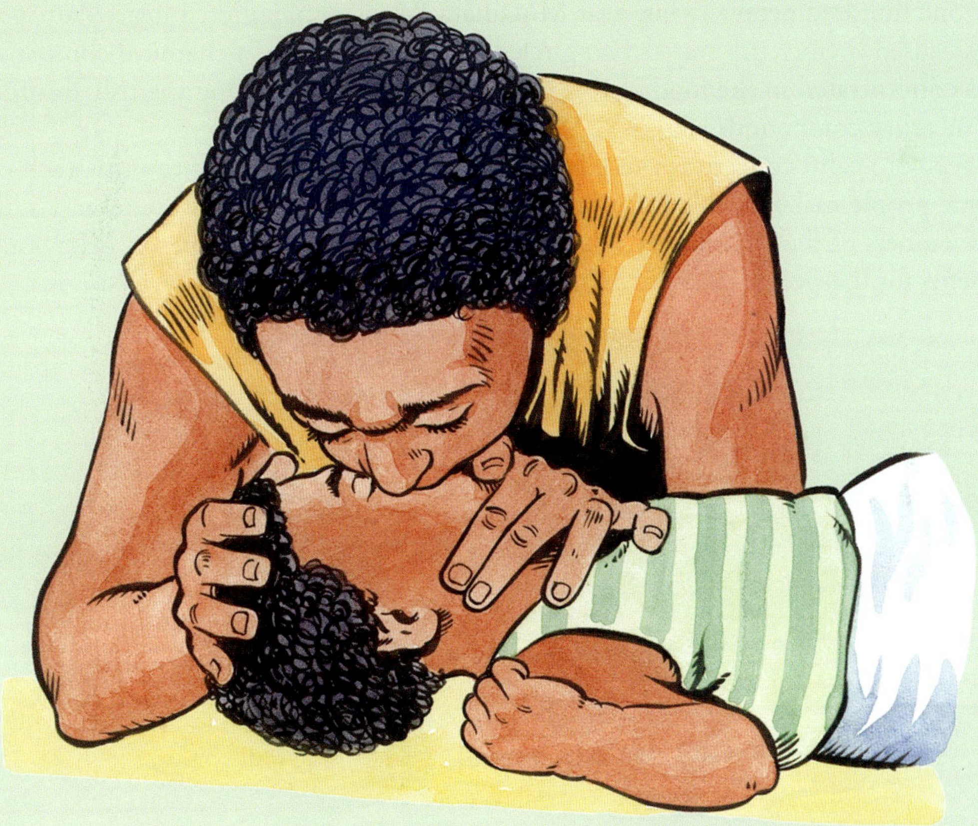

For you to try

- What are the safety rules in your school or community? List them and explain why they are important. If there are no rules then make up a set of rules and give reasons for them. Remember that good rules should be based on common sense and be easy to understand and follow. The number of rules should be kept as small as possible.
- Look for and collect signs and safety symbols that are found in your community or on things that are used in the community. Draw them in your book—put them in groups or categories.

Community health

COMMON HEALTH CONCERNS

There are a number of things that may happen in the community that can affect the health of people. One example is pollution in the environment. Air pollution or smoking can lead to people having breathing problems or lung diseases. Water pollution caused by waste disposal and chemicals that come from factories or mining can spoil water that is used for drinking and affect the fish and shellfish that live in rivers and the sea. Eating fish or shellfish that come from polluted water can make people sick. Many big fish eat smaller fish, so the chemicals can increase or be multiplied further along the **food chain**. Shellfish feed by filtering the water, which has the effect of increasing the chemical pollution and bacteria in the shellfish.

One of the most famous examples of a poison being passed along the food chain happened in Japan. Over one hundred people living near Minamata Bay died or suffered nerve damage. The problem was caused by mercury wastes being released into the bay by a chemical company. The mercury was concentrated in the food chains in the bay, and people eating the fish absorbed large amounts of mercury compounds.

Another type of health concern is caused by the way that people behave towards each other. For example, some people make trouble for others, try to frighten them or treat them very unfairly. Sometimes members of the community refuse to cooperate. All of these types of behaviour can lead to health problems for the people who are being treated wrongly.

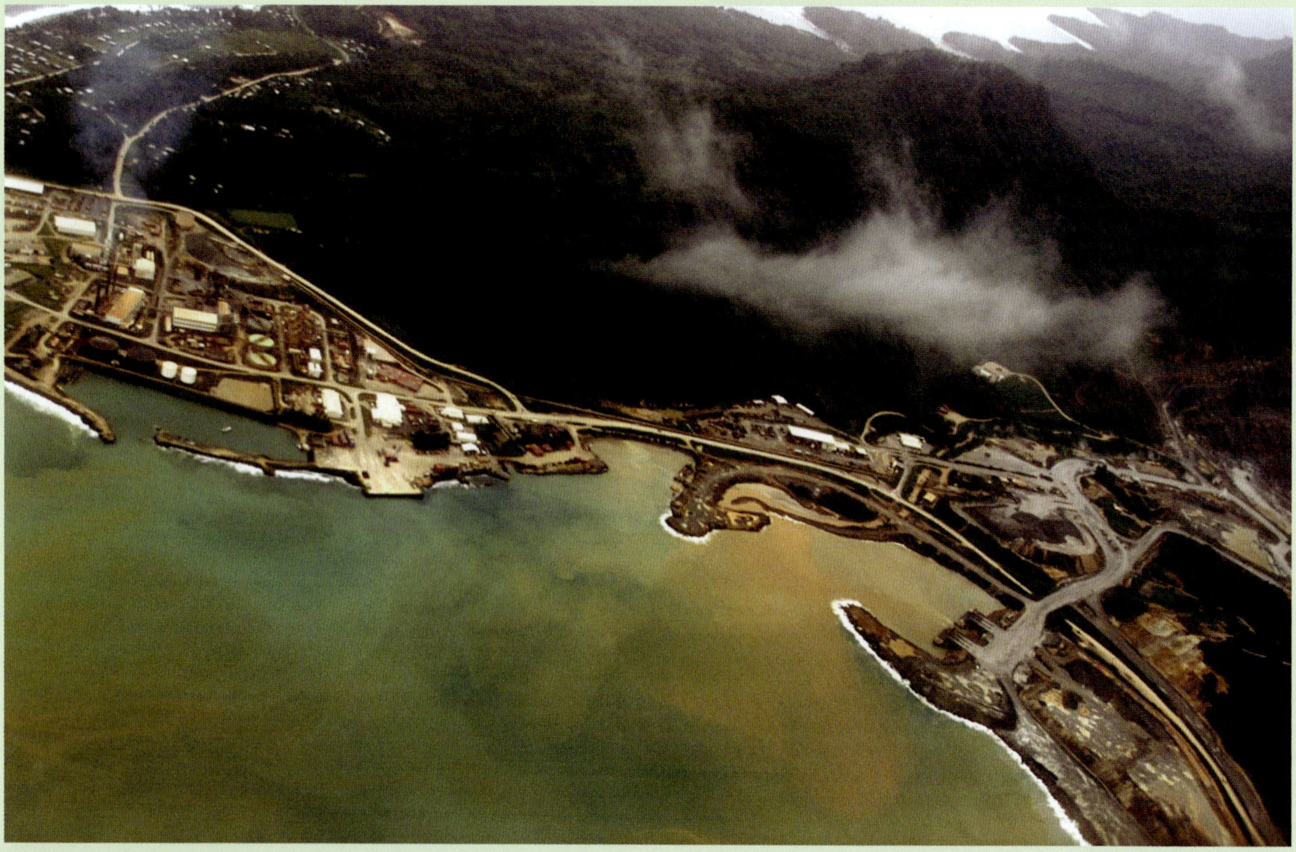

Waste is dumped in the sea from a mine

Ways to help healthy living

The following will all help people to live in healthy ways:

- clean water for drinking and cooking
- keeping water and air pollution as small as possible
- proper waste disposal to get rid of rubbish
- road signs to help drivers and other road users
- safety procedures and policies, such as for the use of small boats in coastal provinces
- cooperation, tolerance and respect among individuals
- celebrating events peacefully

Ways to deal with problems

We sometimes need to look hard for new ways to deal with problems in the community that have been going on for some time. We may need to use more than one way to help to solve a problem. Some of these are:

- Hold meetings between the people involved to discuss the topic.
- Talk with any authority that may be involved.
- Follow rules and policies.
- Dealing with conflict in ways that are acceptable—attack the problem, not the person.
- Suggest changes to rules if this will help with better living.

For you to try

- What are the common health concerns in your community? Make a list.
- Think of one health concern of your community or a community that you know well. Write down some ways to reduce the effect of this health concern.
- Imagine that you are a village councillor. Develop an action plan to deal with health concerns in the community.

FAMILY SIZE

The size of a family has an effect on families and communities. Positive effects of bigger families are:

- The family and community have more people who can do the work that needs to be done.
- There are more people to provide love, care and protection for other members of the family, especially children and old people.
- Members of the family can support each other when something such as food is needed or when a family member needs help.

The negative effects of bigger families are:

- the movement of people from rural to urban areas
- the need for more schools
- economic issues such as finding enough money to pay for school fees and food
- not having enough land, money and food for everyone
- the need for more health services
- greater health risks for mothers and children
- social problems when the needs of people are not met

For you to try

- Carry out a survey to find the size of families of the students in your class. Compare the number of brothers and sisters that you have with the number of brothers and sisters that your parents have. How is it different?
- What is the effect of the increase in the size of the community and population on services and facilities like schools and hospitals in Papua New Guinea?
- Discuss the following topic: Families in Papua New Guinea should have a maximum of two children.
- Write a story giving your views about the size of families in Papua New Guinea and the effect that this will have. Say what you think should happen in the future and give reasons for your point of view.

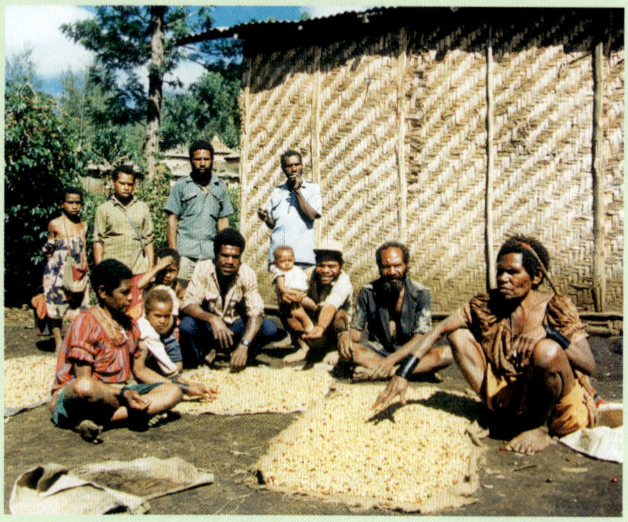

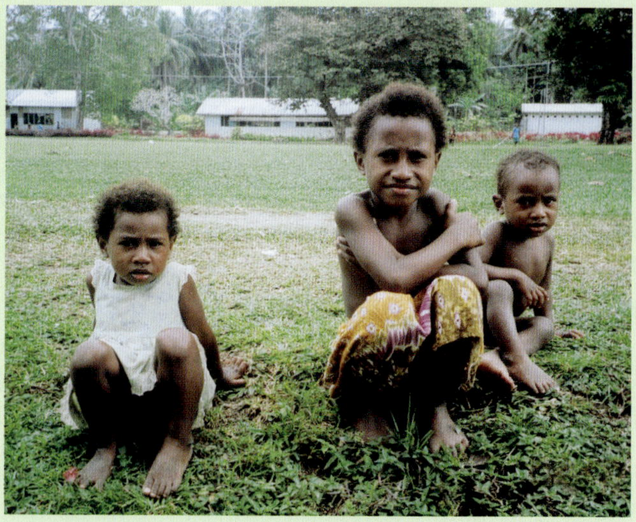

The use of drugs (S)

THE EFFECTS OF DRUG USE ON THE COMMUNITY

When people use drugs there may be a number of effects on the lives of people in the community:

- There may a breakdown in normal family relationships.
- There may be a breakdown in law and order.
- There may be conflict between families, clans and villages.
- Some members of the community may develop poor health.
- Some people may be unable to work.
- Diseases such as STIs and HIV/AIDS will spread more easily.
- The reputation of the community and respect for it will be damaged.

Short-term effects of smoking

When people smoke tobacco there will some short-term effects on their bodies and health:

- Their breath and hair will smell.
- Lung capacity decreases so that they cannot breathe as well.
- The blood carries less oxygen.
- The pulse rate goes up so that the heart is doing more work than it needs to do.
- The activity of the brain increases because it is doing more work than it needs to do.
- The sense of taste and smell decreases.
- The flow of blood to the skin is decreased.
- The level of fitness decreases.
- The temperature of the skin decreases.

Long-term effects of smoking

When people smoke for a long time, there can be serious effects on their health. Smoking causes more sickness in the world than any other reason. Lung diseases such as emphysema, chronic bronchitis, smoker's cough and lung cancer may develop. Smokers may also have other health problems such as heart disease.

In June 2004, the Premier of the state of Tasmania in Australia died of lung cancer. The story was reported in newspapers and on radio and television because of the important message that he sent to everyone.

Premier of Tasmania dies of lung cancer

Shortly before he died of lung cancer on 20 June 2004, the Premier of Tasmania, Jim Bacon, gave a stark health warning: cigarette smoking was for idiots.

'It's a stupid, stupid habit,' Mr Bacon, 53, said. 'I have been a smoker for 35 years . . . I have been an idiot. I have not listened. I have kept smoking. I now accept that I am in large part paying the price for that stupidity.

'The message from me to everyone is please, don't be a fool like me. Don't keep smoking. And if you are young and you haven't started, don't start.'

Possible long-term effects of alcohol

When people drink alcohol over a long period of time there can be a number of serious effects on the health of the drinker, although other people can also be affected. For example:

- violence
- loss of job
- malnutrition
- cancer
- cirrhosis (disease) of the liver
- alcoholism
- brain damage and memory failure

Drinking can become dangerous or harmful when we drink too much, especially for people who drink regularly. Because their bodies are different, women can drink less than men before it becomes dangerous or harmful, as shown in the two tables below:

Standard drinks per day

	Low risk	**Dangerous**	**Harmful**
Male	Fewer than 4	5–6	More than 6
Female	Fewer than 2	3–4	More than 4

Standard drinks per week

	Low risk	**Dangerous**	**Harmful**
Male	Fewer than 28	28–42	More than 42
Female	Fewer than 14	14–28	More than 28

When drinks are bought by the bottle or can, they are not standard drinks. One bottle or can of beer is the same as one-and-a-half standard drinks.

In order to help solve a drinking problem:

- Never drink alone.
- Don't spend your time with people who are heavy drinkers.
- Avoid drinking just after work.
- Avoid drinking in the morning.

For you to try

- What are the reasons why people take legal and illegal drugs?
- List the reasons why tobacco and alcohol are used in Papua New Guinea. Which of these reasons would influence you to take these two drugs?
- Make groups of four or five students. Through a role play, show the effects of too much alcohol, tobacco or other drugs on the behaviour and health of individuals and the community.
- Use the two tables showing the number of standard drinks per day and per week to make two similar tables showing the number of bottles of beer in each of the three categories (low risk, harmful and dangerous) for both males and females.

Programs offered by support agencies

Because drugs can become a big problem in the community, a number of different groups provide help to people using drugs and to their families:

- church groups: family life and drugs
- non-government organisations: community living and productive life
- public health: family life counselling for better health

For you to try

- Find out about groups in your community that help people who have problems or concerns about taking drugs.
- In pairs or groups, discuss how you can help to maintain or establish groups that help other people deal with the problem of drugs in the community. Say what strategies or methods you would use.
- Carry out a community campaign to help people deal with drug problems in the community.

10

Living and Working Together

Chapter Summary

In this chapter you will have an opportunity to:

- ✔ Find out about the choices that we can make when we live in a community
- ✔ Make decisions about a number of issues that occur at school
- ✔ Find out about more about the way that we choose good and fair leaders
- ✔ Find out about the duties and obligations that we all have to keep the laws of the community
- ✔ Discuss the reasons why all people should be allowed to live as they choose, to express their point of view and to move from place to place

Syllabus references

Strand: Living and working together
Sub-strands: Making choices, good and fair leaders, rule of law, respecting rights and freedoms

Outcomes:

8.5.1 Describe choices people make when they take part in the community

8.5.2 Make decisions about school and classroom issues

8.5.3 Analyse the processes of choosing good and fair leaders

8.5.4 Describe what duties and obligations members of the community have in upholding society's laws

8.5.5 Debate the importance and value of the right of all people to freedom of expression, movement and lifestyle

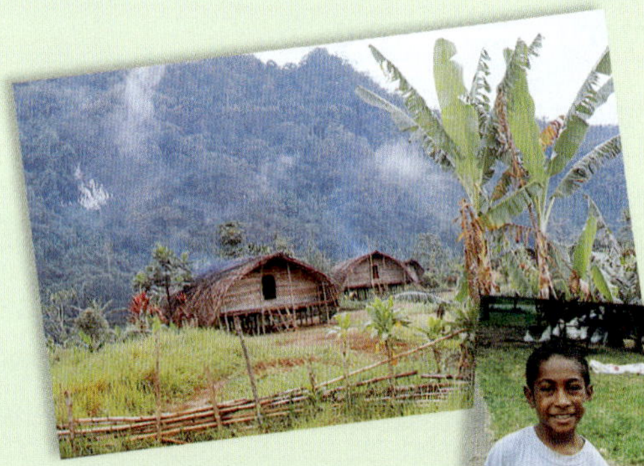

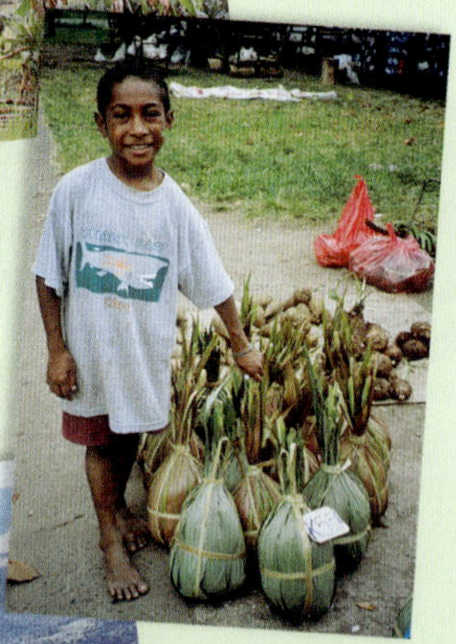

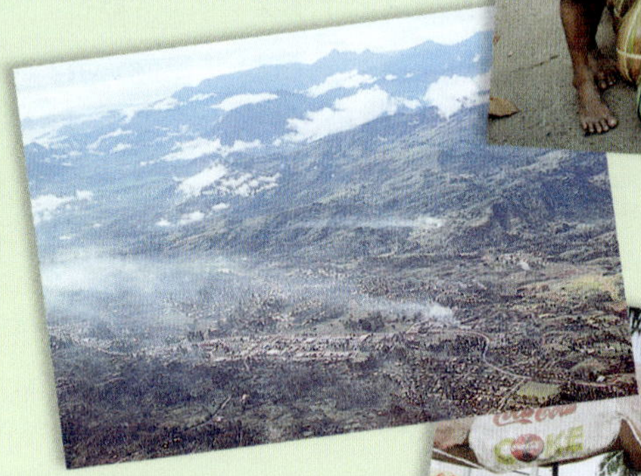

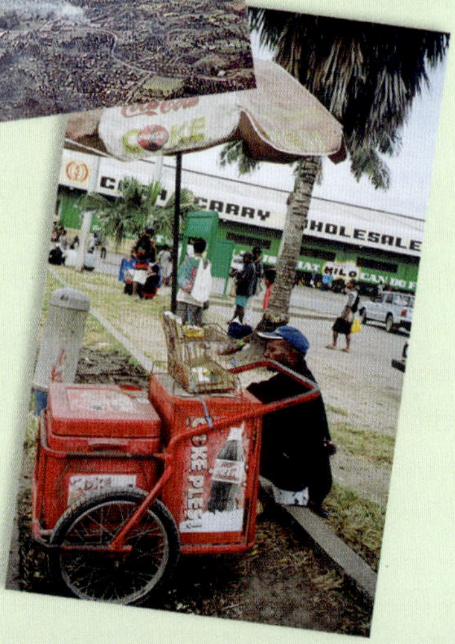

Making choices

POSITIVE CHOICES THAT PEOPLE MAKE

Key facts

- When we take an active part in the community there are many choices to make. Positive attitudes will allow people to make positive choices, but negative actions will discourage free choice.
- Students at school need to make choices about various things that may happen at school and need to find ways to solve problems when they happen.
- There are ways of choosing good and fair leaders and we need to understand the way that this process works.
- All communities have laws and it is the duty of all members of the community to follow the laws and help others to follow them.
- We all have the right and freedom to live as we choose, to express our point of view and to move from place to place.

When we live in a community and take part in the life of the community, there are many choices that we can make in our daily lives. For example, we can choose to be respectful to each other and to live peacefully. We can choose to cooperate with other people and to take part in the life of the community.

As we grow up other young people and adults will look up to us and we can become a role model for other people. Then one day we may be chosen as a leader. Even if we are not chosen as a leader, we can show that we have the qualities of a leader by being a good example for other people to follow, and by being interested in the community and caring about others. Most people want to be accepted in the community, and to do this we need to be open-minded, to share our skills and resources. We need to look after ourselves but also to show commitment to other people in the community.

POSITIVE ATTITUDES

In order to make positive choices, we need to have positive attitudes. When a person has a negative attitude, this affects many of the choices that they make and the things that they do. For example, two people can look at the same thing or the same situation and see two different things, so that a positive person would describe a cup as 'half full' but a negative person would describe it as 'half empty'. A negative person will see the problems and difficulties, but a positive person will see the challenges and the opportunities to achieve something good.

People with positive attitudes often help other people to feel good and help them to achieve the things that they want to achieve. Examples of positive attitudes are:

- being loving and caring
- having a sense of achievement
- working well with others

- being imaginative and innovative—thinking of new ideas and new ways to deal with problems
- having close relationships with other people
- being honest
- assisting others to do what they want to do
- standing up for your beliefs
- participating in different activities
- having a sense of duty to other people
- using authority in a way that shows respect
- respecting other people
- being accountable for your actions
- having pride in what you do so that you do things as well as you can
- being understanding towards other people
- being knowledgeable

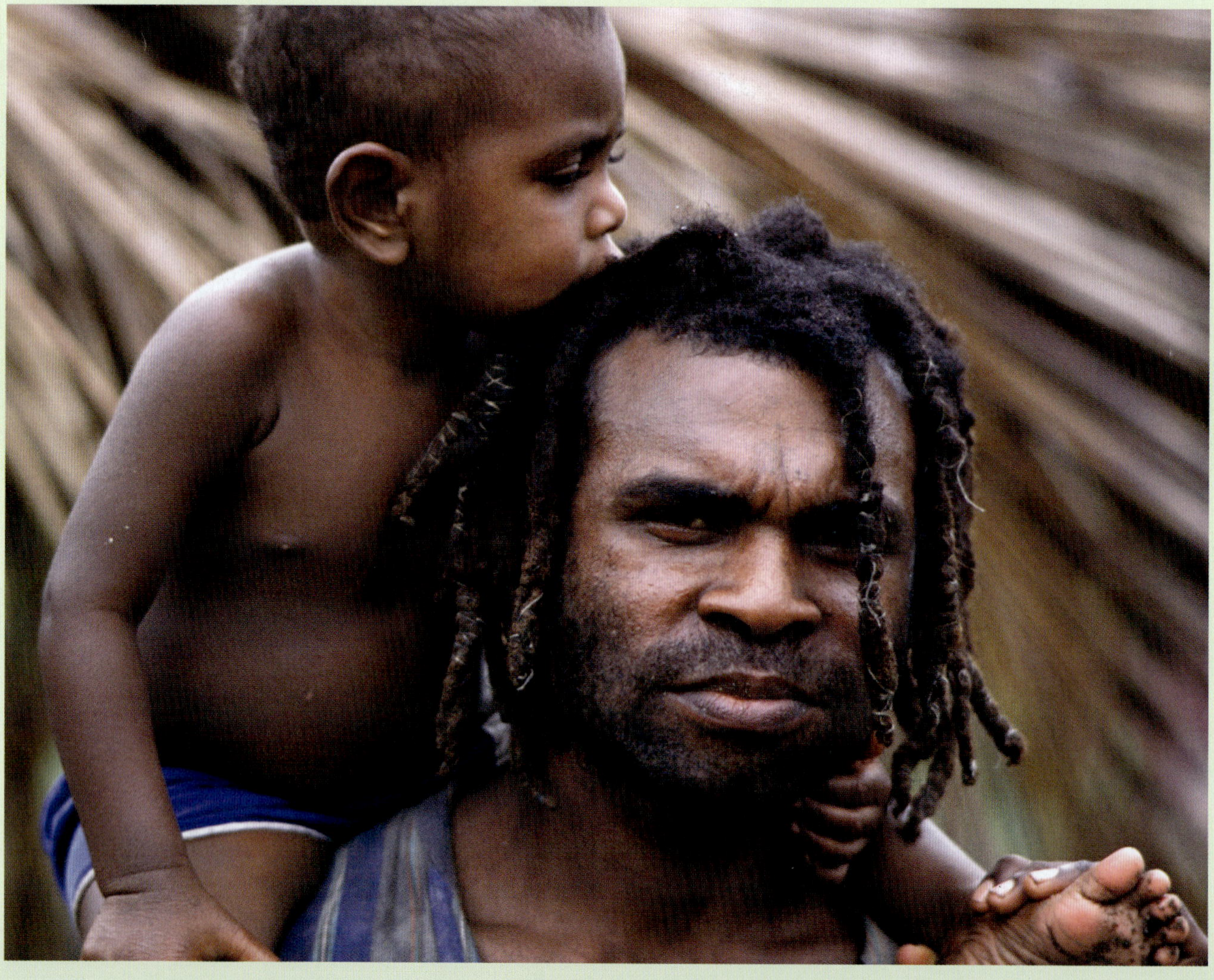

NEGATIVE ACTIONS THAT DISCOURAGE FREE CHOICE

People with negative attitudes often cannot see the possible ways to deal with a problem and may not be very encouraging towards other people when they are trying to do something. Negative attitudes are shown in the following examples:

- working against other people
- not sharing resources in the community
- not taking care of property
- stealing or misusing money that belongs to the community
- talking negatively about other people
- not keeping promises

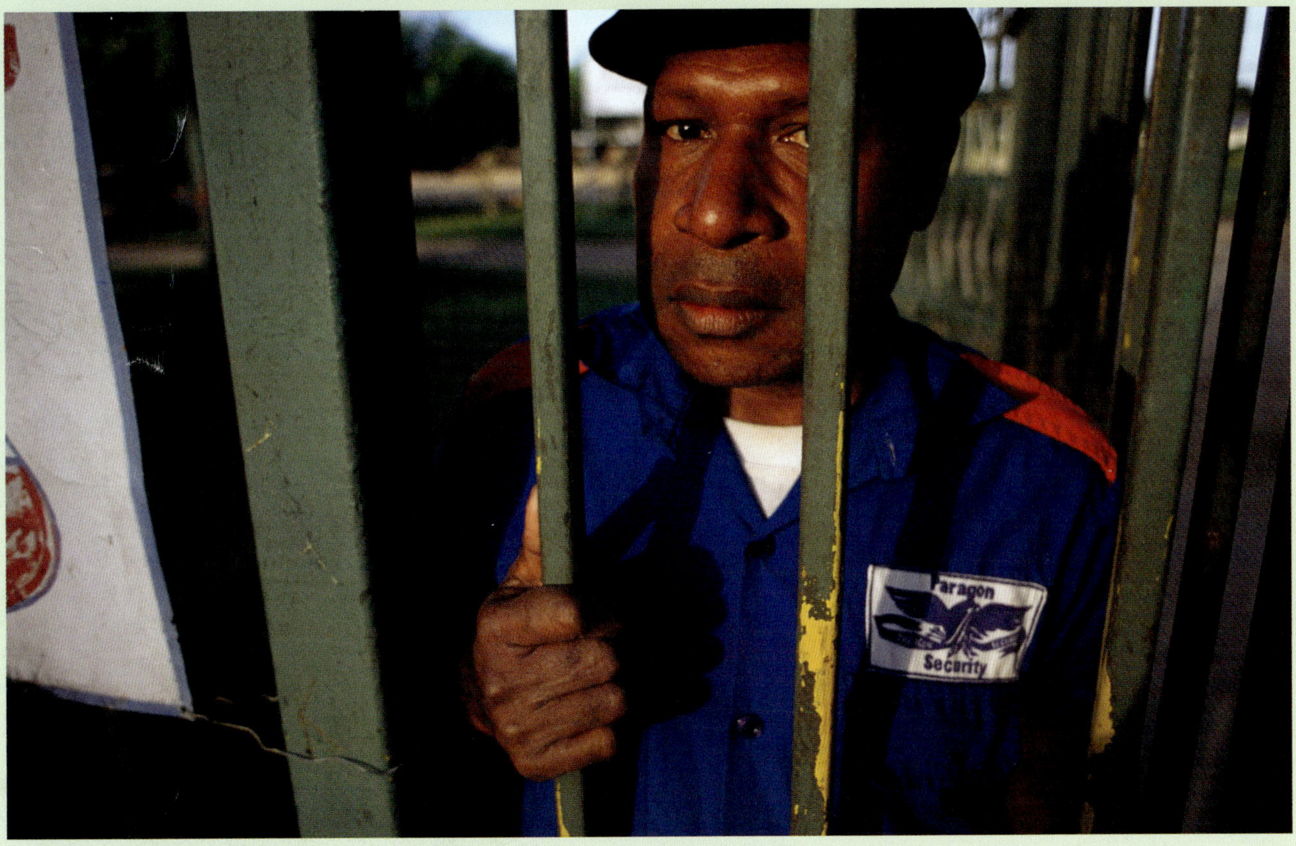

For you to try

- Make groups of four or five students. Discuss the choices that people make when they want to be part of a community group.
- List the influences that affect the choices that people make.
- Describe some of the negative actions that discourage the free choices that people make.

CLASSROOM OR SCHOOL ISSUES

When we are part of a school community there are many choices that we can make in the classroom and generally in the school. If people make poor choices then a number of problems are likely to arise in the school. For example, if people do not respect each other, the following problems may arise:

- teasing, bullying and fighting—making fun of people and trying to make people do things that they do not want to do, or even hitting them or hurting them
- discrimination and equity issues—treating people badly or unfairly because of the place they are from, or because of their gender, or because they are disabled
- showing disrespect for teachers—not listening to them or not doing what they tell you
- problems between boys and girls, especially if they make friends but do not know how to treat each other.

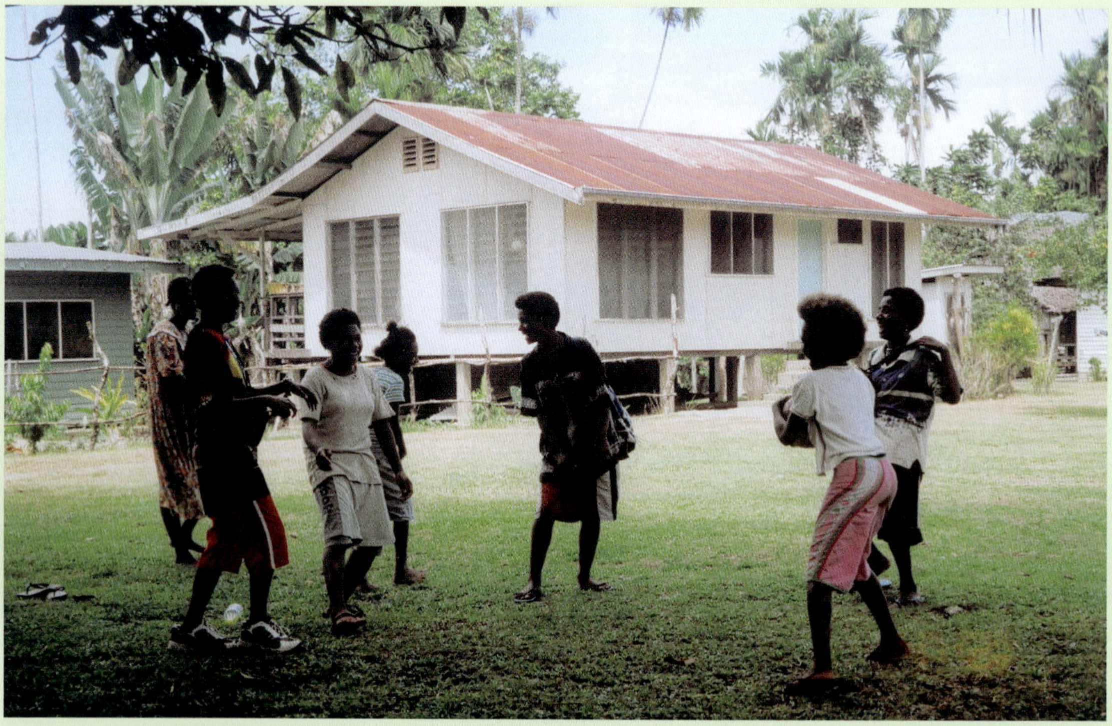

WAYS TO SORT OUT PROBLEMS

There are a number of things that we can do to sort out problems when they arise. Working through problems step-by-step provides a way to approach them each time one arises.

- Firstly, we need to gather information about the problem.
- Secondly, we need to decide what are the causes of the problem.
- Thirdly, we need to suggest solutions to the problem.
- Finally, we need to make a decision about what we will do and carry out the decision.

If we are dealing with a number of issues, then after gathering information we can classify the issues or group them together and deal with similar issues together.

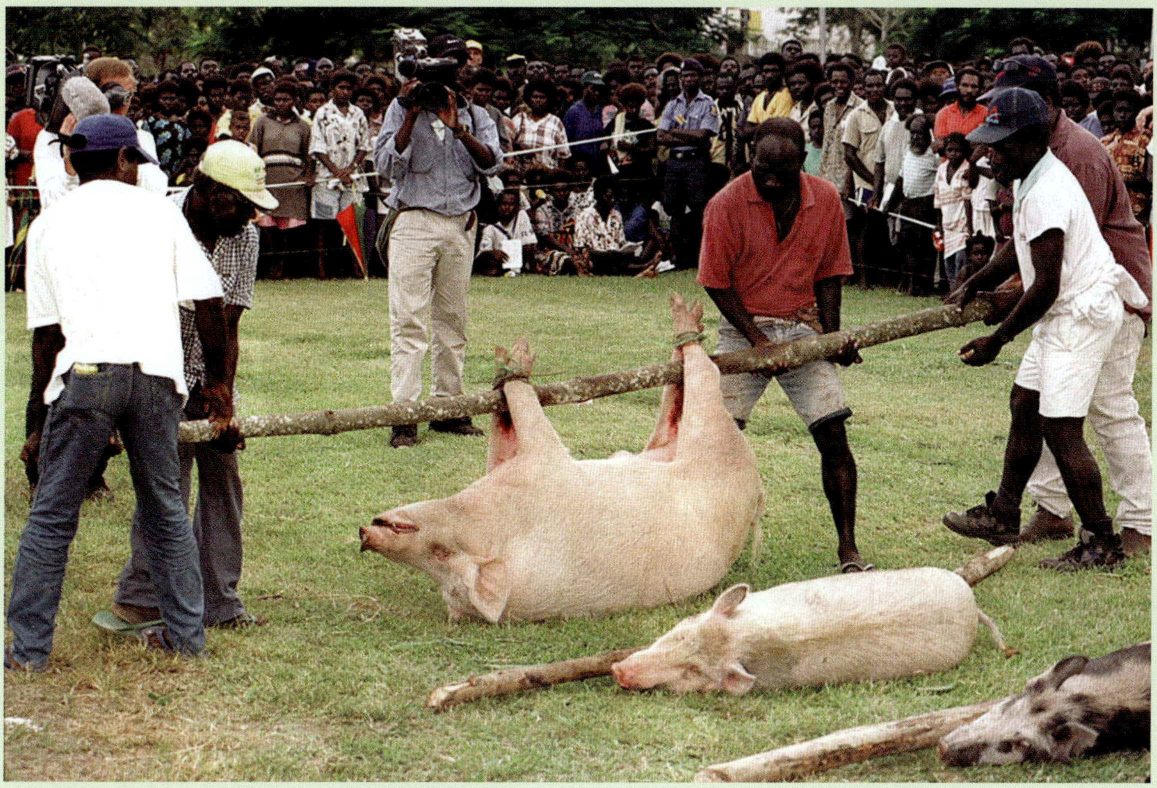

Live pigs offered as a gesture of reconciliation

For you to try

- Talk to different people to find out the issues in your school or community.
  - Make a list of the issues and classify them from the most important to the least important
  - Discuss and describe the causes of these problems.
  - What can individuals and the community do in order to solve these problems?
- Role play a situation in which there is bullying in school and how to deal with that situation.

Good and fair leaders

CHOOSING LEADERS

People in different communities choose leaders in different ways. For example, in **traditional societies** people listened to the elders and respected what they said. Many leaders were older men although in some societies women also had an important position. In some societies leaders were was chosen because they came from a particular clan, or because they were very wealthy. Sometimes people were chosen because of their family relationships or because they were the most educated people in the community.

In **modern societies** there is a way for choosing or electing leaders that is accepted by people in many parts of the world. This method can be used by students in school, by people in sports clubs or church groups, and by a province or a country to choose political leaders.

The first step is to call for **nominations**. This means that someone suggests that the **candidate** should stand for election. A candidate is a person who can be elected. Usually somebody else nominates the candidate and the candidate then has to agree to stand for election, although in some elections the candidate can nominate himself or herself.

The next step is put the names of all the candidates on a piece of paper called a **ballot paper**. The people taking part in the election can then choose the person or the people that they want by marking the ballot paper. In an election to choose leaders the people are called **voters**, because when people make their choice they are 'voting' for that person. Each person should be able to vote for the person that they think is best without being influenced by anyone else. The ballot or election should also be secret so that no one else knows how you voted. Then if someone asks how you voted, you do not have to tell him or her.

The final step in an election is to count the votes and find out who the winner is. Usually, the person who has the most votes is the winner. This is sometimes called '**first past the post**'.

In 2004 a new system called **Limited Preferential Voting** was introduced in Papua New Guinea for national elections. Voters must vote '1, 2, 3' for their first, second and third choices. A candidate can only be declared the winner when they have an absolute majority, which means more than half of the votes counted. All the number ones, or voters' first choices, are counted. If no one has reached an absolute majority, then the candidate with the lowest number of votes is removed and the second choices are given to the remaining candidates and counted. If no one has reached an absolute majority, the next candidate with the least number of votes is again removed and the process repeated until there is a candidate with more than half the votes counted.

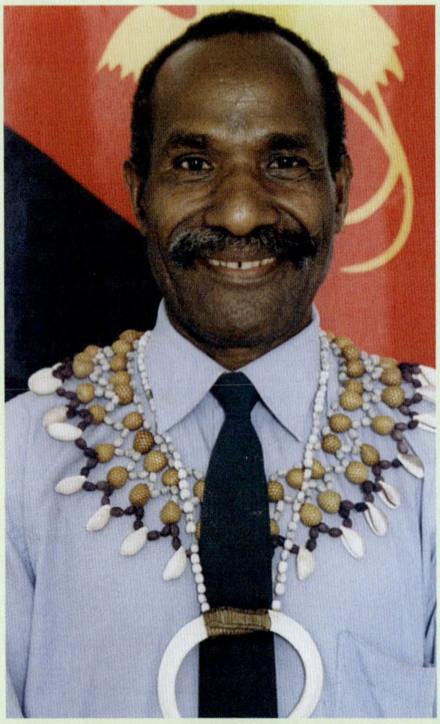

A candidate in the 2002 elections

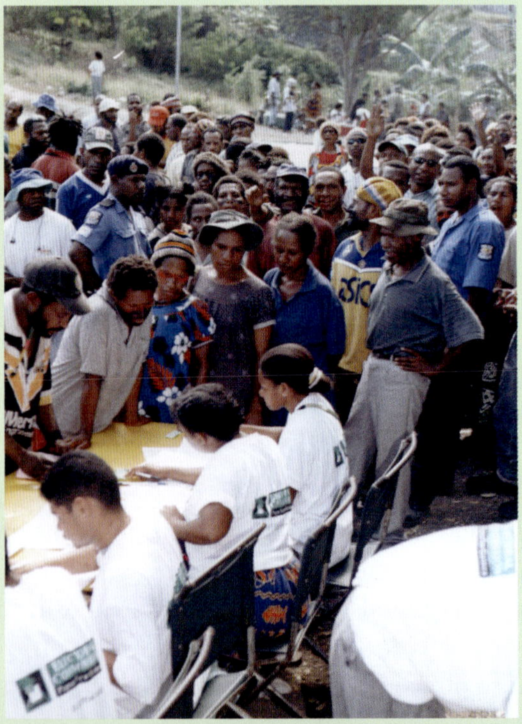

People line up to vote in the 2002 elections

When we elect Members of Parliament the candidates give speeches, make promises and meet the people. This is called an **election campaign**. The campaign and the voting process should be fair and no one should do anything dishonest to help one candidate win.

On election day everyone who has his or her name on the electoral roll or list can vote and the voters put their ballot papers in a locked box. The ballot boxes are then taken to a **tally room** where the votes are counted. The candidates with an absolute majority or more than half the votes counted are the winners and represent their province or district as Members of Parliament in the National Government.

WAYS TO HELP US CHOOSE GOOD LEADERS

When we choose leaders there are a number of things that we can do in order to help the process to work well. For example:

- We should listen to what other people have to say before making a decision.
- We should choose the person with the best ideas and skills to be a leader.
- Voters should not be threatened but feel free to make their own choice.
- When people try to force us to vote for somebody that we do not want to vote for, we should not give in to them.
- We should choose a candidate who has a reputation for being honest and well-informed.
- We should not accept money or other goods in order to vote for a particular person—this is called bribery.
- We should choose a leader who is healthy, wise and energetic. People who are not healthy, not sensible and do not have energy will find it very difficult to be a good leader.
- We should expect a high standard of moral and ethical principles from our elected leaders. They should know what is right and follow the right way.

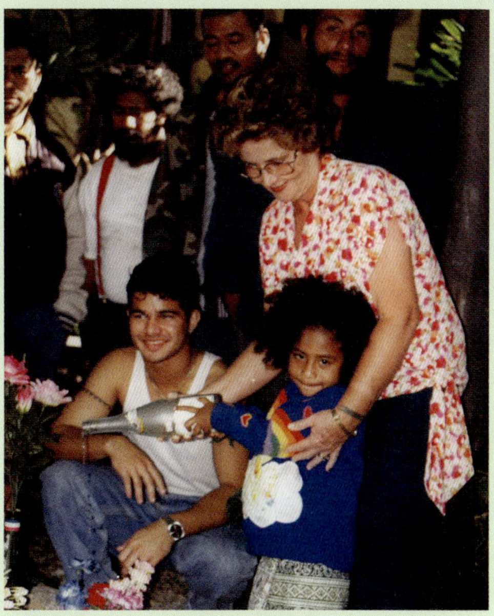

Lady Carol Kidu, cabinet minister

For you to try

- What are the different ways that we can choose a leader? How are leaders chosen in your school or in your community?
- A How are political leaders chosen in your province and for Papua New Guinea? Who are the provincial politicians and national politicians in your area?
- Give a two-minute talk to the class to explain how the ways of choosing leaders could be improved.
- Identify a national or community leader who has helped your community. Discuss how to support this leader to improve the community.

Rules and laws

KEEPING THE LAWS

All communities have rules and laws which show people the way that they should behave and make it easier for people to live together in the community.

The rules and laws that we have in a country help to give us our **rights**. They also give us **responsibilities**. For example, we have the right to feel safe, to vote for our leaders and to belong to any church, but we do not have the right to take things that belong to other people. If everyone did what they wanted to do without thinking about other people, then there would be a lot of trouble in the community. So we must also consider other people. We say that we all have the right to do as we please as long as we do not take away the rights of other people.

Our responsibilities are the things that we must do in order to follow the law and be a good citizen and a useful member of the community. Responsibilities are sometimes known as **duties** and **obligations**. All people have certain responsibilities, but some people have special responsibilities because of their position. Some of the responsibilities of citizens and leaders are as follows:

Citizens

- obey and respect the laws of the country
- feed and care for other people
- support and assist in the education of children
- respect and care for the environment
- create a stable family life

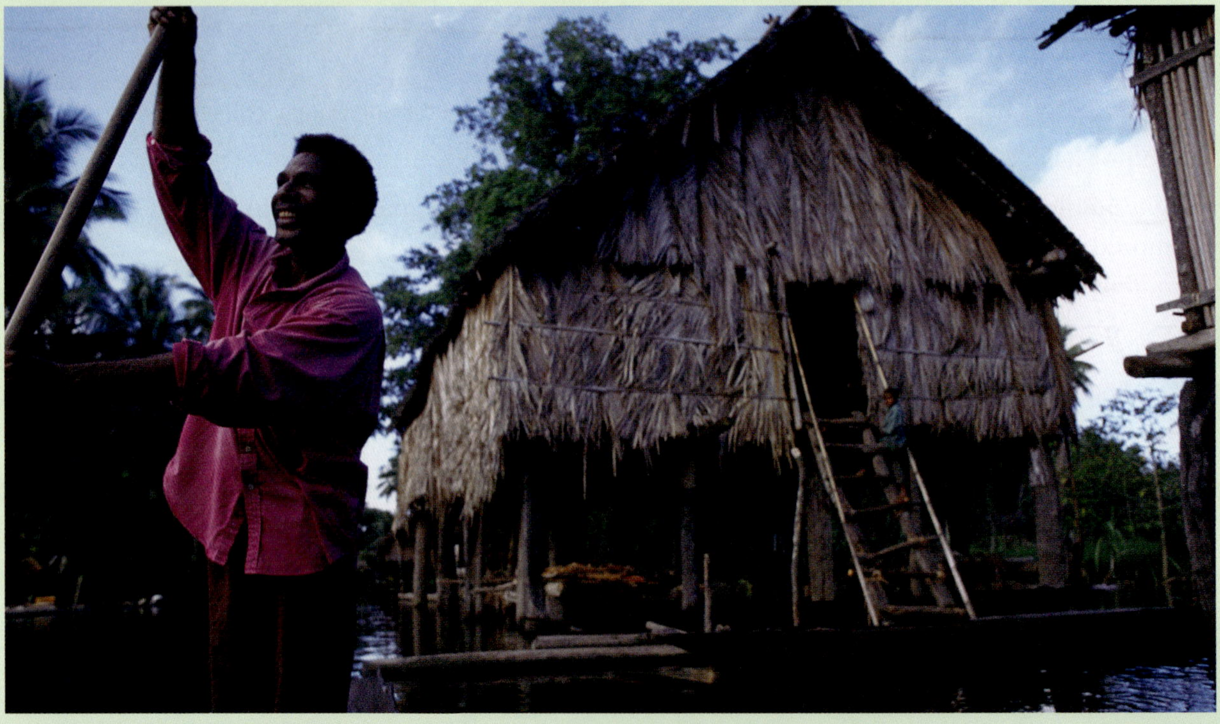

Leaders

- obey and respect the laws of the country
- help to make sure that other people follow the laws
- help to solve problems in the community
- support members of the community in their beliefs, such as their spiritual or religious life
- provide advice or counselling to people who need it
- act as a good role model for other people in the community to follow

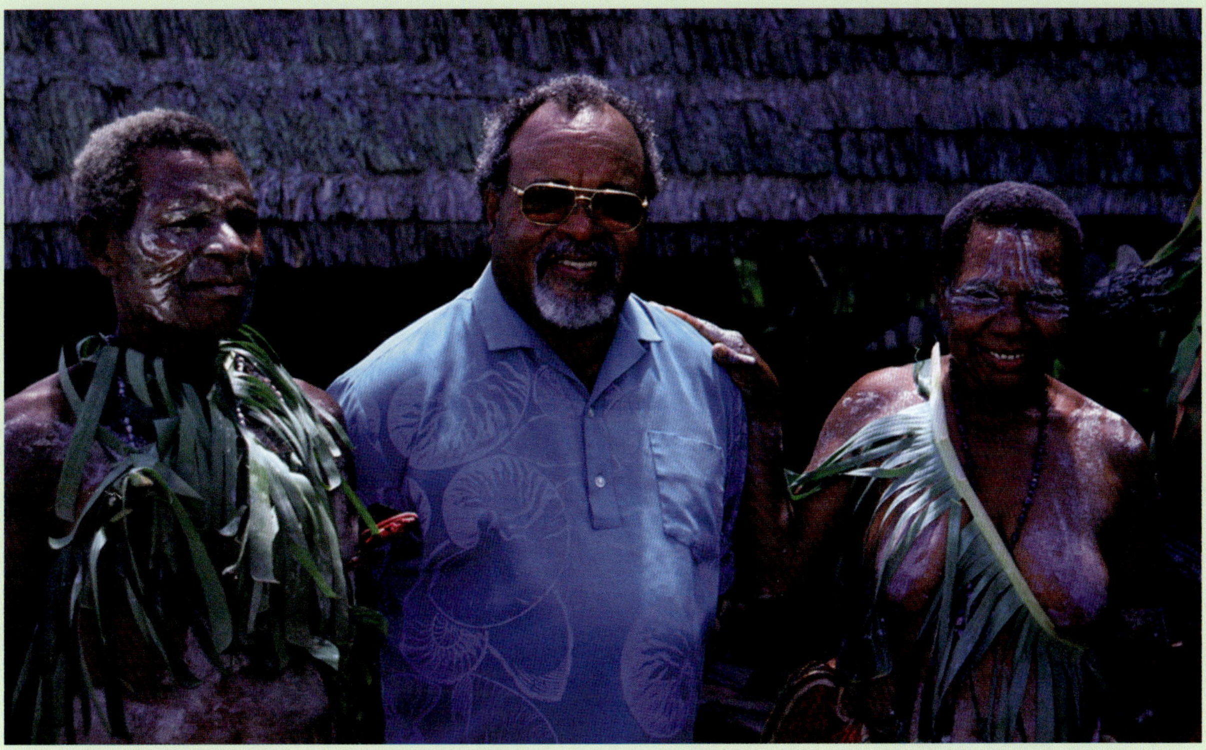

Sir Michael Somare, Prime Minister of Papua New Guinea, with people from the Middle Sepik region

For you to try

A Make groups of three or four students and discuss the differences between rights and responsibilities. Make two lists of examples like the one below:

Rights	Responsibilities

For you to try

- Look at the following list of rights and responsibilities:

	Right	Responsibility
Voting in an election		
Travelling freely and safely from place to place		
Paying for the registration of a car		
Following the religion that you choose		
Looking after children		
Going to school for as long as you like		

Copy and complete the table and say which are rights, which are responsibilities and which are both.

- In groups of four or five students, discuss and describe how people can support the rules and laws of their community.
- Explain the advantages and disadvantages of observing or not observing rules and laws.

Respecting rights and freedoms

All people have rights and freedoms that should be respected. We expect to have these rights for ourselves and we also need to let other people have their rights and freedoms.

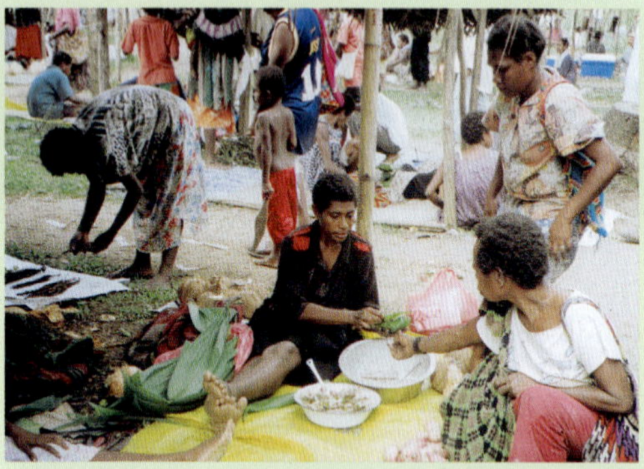

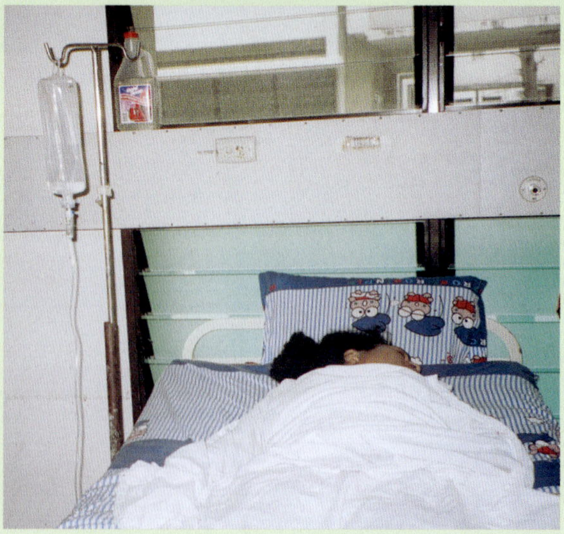

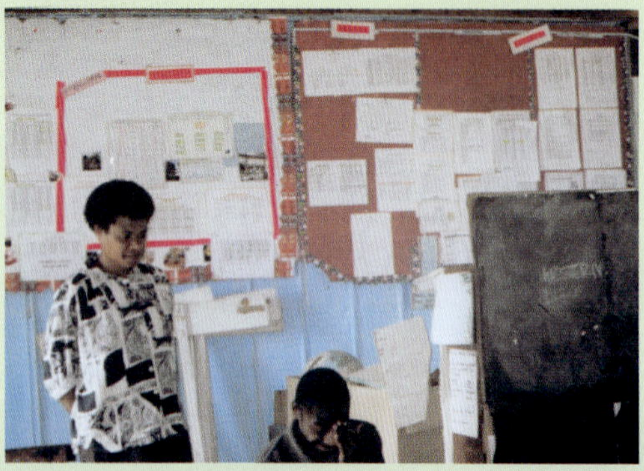

Your Rights

Freedom of expression and speech—to talk freely using different media and to give our own ideas on any topic, such as religion or politics. People should be able to speak any language they choose.

The right to vote for leaders—to choose the person we think is the best for the position without being forced or influenced by anyone else.

Freedom of movement and assembly—to move from place to place within and outside Papua New Guinea and to hold meetings with other people. People should be able to go anywhere at any time.

Freedom from discrimination. No one should treat people unfairly because of things like the place they are from, the group that they belong to, or their gender. People should also be able to express their sexuality freely.

Freedom of choice of lifestyle—so that each person can live in the way that they choose to live. People should also be able to live and work in any place they choose.

The right to education—so that every person can have the opportunity to go to both primary and secondary school to complete their education.

The right to health and welfare services—so that everyone can get medical care and treatment. This should include immunisations for children and pregnant women that help to prevent sickness.

For you to try

- Choose one of the rights mentioned above.
  - Write a short report to say why this right is important and why you value it.
  - Suggest ways to promote standards of behaviour that promote or encourage this right.

Additional Projects and Investigations

GRADE 7

Chapter 1: Relationships

1 Write down the family tree for your family or work out the family tree for a well-known family.

2 Find out more about different kinds of families in other countries.

3 Invite an older person to come to the school to talk to the students about family life in previous times. What was the place of children and grandparents? How did people choose a husband or wife? How were things different then?

If possible, ask them to show you some of things that people used years ago in their homes or in their work, or to show you some old pictures or old papers. Remember that we need to be careful with old things because they can sometimes easily be broken.

4 Using the words in the list, find the words that are missing from the passage below. You can use each word only once.

skills countries family families different similarities role

We are all members of a family although there are many different types of ____________________. Families can be ____________________ in the same country and can also be different in other ____________________ in the world. People play different roles in each ____________________ and there is an accepted code of behaviour for each relationship and group. People can be described by their ____________________ to and differences from each other. People take on different roles in a family. When we take on a particular ____________________, this affects our relationships, attitude and behaviour. Relationships are important in families and ____________________ are needed to maintain effective relationships.

5 Which of the following are provided by all families?
A. housing
B. food
C. clothing

(a) A only
(b) B only
(c) A and B only
(d) A, B and C

6 Which of the following are usually provided by all families?
A. respect
B. comfort
C. love
D. security

(a) A and B only
(b) B and C only
(c) A, B and C
(d) A, B, C and D

7 Which of the following do we need to learn to do in our relationships?
A. Make good decisions about the things that we do
B. Develop respect for other people
C. Feel positive about ourselves but not other people

(a) C only
(b) A and B only
(c) B and C only
(d) A, B and C

8 Which of the following do we need to learn to do in our relationships?
A. Recognise the needs of other people
B. Ignore the opinions of other people
C. Develop positive values like being trustworthy, helpful and sharing
D. Be assertive and confident to say what we think

(a) A, B and D only
(b) B, C and D only
(c) A, C and D only
(d) A, B, C and D

9 Which of the following do parents usually want their children to do?
A. Behave in ways that are acceptable to the family or group
B. Know what behaviour is expected at different times and places
C. Understand the reasons why we behave in certain ways
D. Always ask parents to make decisions for them

(a) A and B only
(b) B and C only
(c) A, B and C only
(d) A, B, C and D

10 When we deal with problems that we have with other people, we need to:
A. Hide our feelings from other people
B. Give our point of view without getting angry or fighting
C. Learn what to do when other people get angry

(a) A and B only
(b) B and C only
(c) A and C only
(d) A, B and C

11 Which of the following best describes people who belong to the same group?
A. Often have the same interests and values, and carry out similar activities
B. Often share the same interests but have very different values and activities
C. Often wear similar dress or have similar appearance but different values
D. Sometimes have the same diet but usually follow different activities

12 Which of the following are ways that we learn to be a member of a group and to share the same values?
A. Copying other members of the group
B. Being told by others and asking questions
C. Following the traditions of the group
D. Telling other members of the group when you disagree with them

(a) A, B and D only
(b) A, C and D only
(c) A, B and C only
(d) A, B, C and D

13 Which of the following are ways that are most likely to maintain effective relationships with other people?
A. Listen carefully to others and respect what they say
B. Speak firmly to people when they make mistakes
C. Think positively about yourself and others
D. Tell other people what is happening when they need to know

(a) A, B and D only
(b) A, B and C only
(c) A, C and D only
(d) A, B, C and D

14 Which of the following are likely to happen when a relationship starts to break down and people feel like fighting?

A. Cooperating with each other and listening to each other
B. Getting angry and shouting at each other
C. Deliberately making trouble
D. Trying to shame other people

(a) A, B and C only
(b) A, B and D only
(c) B, C and D only
(d) A, B, C and D

15 Make a table like the one below and list the roles and responsibilities of the people in your family.

Person	Roles and responsibilities
Grandparents	
Parents	
Uncles	
Aunts	
Cousins	
Brothers	
Sisters	

Chapter 2: Movement and Physical Activity

1 Organise a novelty sports day at your school to celebrate the end of term or a special day. Possible events are:

- Egg and spoon race—you can use any round object like betel nuts instead of eggs. (If you have a plastic spoon, try carrying it in your mouth instead of your hand.)
- Sack race—use copra sacks or coffee sacks
- Wheelbarrow race—one person 'walks' along on her hands while her legs are supported by her partner
- Three-legged race—two people tie two of their legs together with a strip of cloth
- Carrying balloons filled with water between the knees
- Hoopla—throw wire rings over a tin or bottle.
- Throwing balls in the bucket—you can make your own balls from coconut leaves or rolling up a number of plastic shopping bags and tying them together.
- Pushing a bar of soap up a slippery slope with a stick
- A slow bicycle race—if you have only two bicycles you can have heats
- Tunnel ball

2 Learn how to give first aid when it is needed. If you do not know how to give first aid, then invite someone to come to the school to teach you.

3 Ask your teacher to invite someone to come to your school to teach self-defence.

4 Carry out a survey to find out about the need for leisure and recreation activities in your school or community. Use a record sheet like the one below.

Leisure activity or recreation	How could this be organised? (Who? Where? When?)	What is needed to make this activity happen?

Make a summary of your findings and tell the rest of the class.

5 Help to organise some 'keeping fit' activities for particular groups in the community.

6 Plan and carry out a mini-sports competition for children in your community. Do this to help celebrate an important day like Independence Anniversary, your provincial day or Christmas Day.

7 Learn and perform some traditional dancing to celebrate an important day like Independence Anniversary, your provincial day or the end of the school year. You will need to plan and practise for some weeks before the event. People from the local community could be invited to teach the dances and to take part in the celebration.

8 Using the words in the list, find the words that are missing from the passage below. You can use each word only once.

people   movements   different   roles   activities   emergencies   dangerous   plans

To take part in games, sports and dance we need to link a range of ____________________ skills together. Skills often involve sequences of movements. When we learn sequences of ____________________, we need to develop good body control. Taking part in a variety of physical ____________________ helps to develop different parts of our fitness. Some sporting activities can be ____________________ and we need to know how to deal with dangerous situations and with ____________________. People are sometimes slow to take part in recreational and leisure activities, and in order to encourage them to take part, suitable ____________________ are needed. Many different ____________________ can be involved in organising sports. In some games and in organised sport, there are different codes of behaviour for the various ____________________ that people take.

9 Which of the following activities involve locomotor skills in which the person moves or travels from place to place?

A. Running, jumping, hopping and skipping combined together
B. Taking off and landing using one foot or two feet
C. Swimming using different arm and leg actions
D. Dancing by standing in one spot and moving the head and upper body

(a) A, B and C only
(b) A, B and D only
(c) B, C and D only
(d) A, B, C and D

Questions 10, 11 and 12 refer to the following information about movement skills.

A. Throw for speed, distance, accuracy and height
B. Move to catch a ball or other object
C. Balance on different parts of the body
D. Perform set body actions in time to rhythm or music
E. Turn or twist correctly during a body movement

10 Which of the skills A–E require body control?

(a) A and B only
(b) C and D only
(c) C, D and E only
(d) A, B, C, D and E

11 Which of the skills are most likely to be used in dance but not sport?
(a) A and B only
(b) C and D only
(c) C, D and E only
(d) A, B, C, D and E

12 Which two skills are most likely to be used in netball, basketball and softball?
(a) A and B
(b) B and C
(c) C and D
(d) D and E

13 Which of the following best describes the sequence of events that you would follow in order to deal with danger such as a fight?
A. If fighting starts, do not stay in that place, especially when it feels unsafe.
B. Report fighting to someone that you trust.
C. If it is safe to do so, go back to help someone who is hurt.
D. Have a plan to avoid risk and carry out your plan.

(a) A, B, C, D
(b) B, D, C, A
(c) D, C, B, A
(d) D, A, B, C

14 Which of the following are good rules to follow in order to help someone who is hurt?
A. Learn how to give first aid so you can help when needed.
B. If you cannot help the person, go and get help from somebody else.
C. Never think of your own safety when helping someone else.

(a) A only
(b) A and B only
(c) B and C only
(d) A, B and C

15 Which of the following are good ways to encourage the whole community to take part in leisure and recreation?
A. Organise activities for people who do not normally take part such as young children, girls and women.
B. Organise activities for fun, not just for winning.
C. Find ways that people can accept losing competitions without getting angry.

(a) A only
(b) A and B only
(c) B and C only
(d) A, B and C

Chapter 3: Our Culture, Lifestyle and Values

1 Visit a site near your school where there have been many changes. Identify and list the changes. Which changes are positive and which are negative?

2 Invite elders from the community to come and talk about the changes that they have noticed in the environment. Which changes do they feel happy about and which changes do they feel unhappy about? What can people do about the changes that are not good changes?

3 Find out about the physical, social and economic changes that have taken place in other places and note the causes for those changes.

4 Using the words in the list, find the words that are missing from the passage below. You can use each word only once.

changes different country life traditions forgotten

Customs, rituals and ____________________ are still strong in Papua New Guinea, but some may be lost or ____________________. There are many differences in the culture of people from ____________________ parts of the country. We should respect our own culture and that of people from other parts of the ____________________ and from other countries. As Papua New Guinea develops, many ____________________ are taking place to the way of ____________________ of people, and some of these are affecting the culture.

Questions 5 and 6 refer to the following list of celebrations.

A. Independence Anniversary
B. Easter
C. Christmas
D. Queen's Birthday
E. New Year's Day

5 Which of the following shows the celebrations A–E in the correct order as they occur, starting at the beginning of the year?
(a) E, A, B, D, C
(b) B, A, D, C, E
(c) E, B, D, A, C
(d) E, D, B, A, C

6 Which are most likely to be celebrated by people in church?
(a) A and B
(b) B and C
(c) B and D
(d) C and D

7 Answer true or false to the following statements about changes that are happening to our way of life.
  a Roads allow people to move about more easily, to buy and sell goods and to reach schools and hospitals.
  b New food crops and farming methods decrease the variety of food available.
  c New cash crops allow people to earn money.
  d Electricity for lights and cooking is important to help keep people healthy.
  e A reliable water supply makes life easier and helps to keep people healthy.
  f Closing of Aid Posts can affect the health of the community.
  g Clearing land for logging or mining can cause damage to land, rivers and wildlife, and loss of farming land.

Questions 8–10 refer to the following changes:

A. Damage to the environment caused by mining or logging
B. Earning money from new cash crops
C. Electricity to allow students to study at night
D. Having a clean water supply and flush toilets

8 Which of the changes A–D are mainly *physical* changes?
(a) A
(b) B
(c) C
(d) D

9 Which of the changes A–D are mainly *economic* changes?
(a) A
(b) B
(c) C
(d) D

10 Which of the changes A–D are mainly *social* changes?
(a) A and C
(b) B and C
(c) B and D
(d) C and D

Chapter 4: Health of Individuals and Population

1 Write down a question about growth and development on a piece of paper. Do not put your name on the paper. Put the paper in a box. Later on your teacher will go through the questions and sort them out. Your teacher will read out each question and talk about the answers with the class.

2 Invite a guest speaker from the community to talk about local customs and rules related to food.

3 Make a plan for the sale of healthy food on special occasions like Independence Anniversary and end of year celebrations. Carry out your plan.

4 In your class or your school, plan and carry out a long-term project to improve the environment of the school or community. For example:
- Plant fruit trees around the school or community.
- Plant shade trees around the school or community.
- Start a nursery for fruit trees and shade trees.
- Build better toilets.
- Organise better rubbish disposal.
- Construct better drains.

Parents and citizens could get involved in such a project.

5 Choose a health problem in your school or in the community. Plan some simple activities that can be used to help people to behave in ways that are more healthy. Show your plans to the other students and your teacher. Choose the best ideas and put them into practice.

6 Invite someone from the Health Department to come and talk about the health problems and social problems that can happen when people take drugs.

7 If students in your class have missed out on vaccinations, your teacher may organise a visit to the local health centre or hospital.

8 Using the words in the list, find the words that are missing from the passages below. You can use each word only once.

illness	appearance	plan	alcohol	community	behave
choices	negative	reproductive	food	drugs	effect

The main purpose of the ____________________ system is to allow men and women to have children. When we grow up from girls into women and from boys into men, many changes take place in our ____________________ and in the way that we feel and behave. The way that we ____________________ can increase or reduce the respect that we have for each other.

Eating is a behaviour that varies in people from different places. People eat different kinds of ____________________ and eat in different ways. Everyone can ____________________ healthy and nutritious meals using food that is available locally.
We can make plans and ____________________ about our own health using our knowledge about what makes us sick. We can keep ourselves healthy by avoiding ____________________ and other risky situations that threaten our personal health and safety. Our behaviour should not have a negative effect on the health of other people in the ____________________. We can also help others in the community to learn about health and safety and to prevent ____________________.

Because of the ways that we live, we are having an effect on the environment, which in turn is having an ____________________ on our health. Drugs can also affect the health of people who use them and have a ____________________ effect on other people in the community. Each person has a choice about whether he or she will use drugs and ____________________.

9 Answer true or false to the following statements.

- **a** The stage in life when you develop into an adult is called puberty.
- **b** Adolescence begins before puberty.
- **c** Puberty usually begins in boys about two years before girls.
- **d** Having periods is a normal thing that happens to every girl.
- **e** When boys and girls grow up, they become taller and heavier and hair begins to grow under the arm and in the pubic area.
- **f** When a boy starts to produce sperm, it is possible for him to become a father.
- **g** When a girl starts to have periods, it is possible for her to become a mother.

10 Fertilisation occurs when the sperm meets the egg:

A. in the vagina
B. in the uterus
C. in the Fallopian tube
D. in the ovaries

11 Fertilisation is also known as:

A. conception
B. contraception
C. family planning
D. sexual intercourse

12 What are the similarities between girls having a period and boys having a wet dream?

A. A liquid comes out of the body.
B. It usually happens regularly.
C. It only happens after puberty has begun.

(a) A only
(b) A and B only
(c) A and C only
(d) A, B and C

13 Answer true or false to the following statements about the social changes that are likely to happen to young people during adolescence.
   a You develop values, beliefs and behaviour that may be influenced by traditional ideas about what it means to be a man or a woman.
   b You become less closely involved with friends or peers.
   c You experiment with new types of relationships, like having a boyfriend or girlfriend.
   d You develop a sense of your own sexuality—the way that you think and feel and behave as a young man or young woman.
   e You become more dependent on other people.

14 Answer true or false to the following statements about the emotional changes that are likely to happen to young people during adolescence.
   a You may have very strong likes and dislikes about people and things.
   b You may feel very aggressive and want to argue with people.
   c You may have strong ideals and views about the way that things should be or the way that other people behave.
   d You may become very critical of other people and get into arguments very easily.

15 In the following list, put a tick in the appropriate column to show which behaviour encourages respect and which reduces respect.

Behaviour	**Encourages respect**	**Reduces respect**
Shouting or using bad language		
Greeting someone by smiling and shaking hands		
Interrupting other people and not letting them give their point of view		
Being humble and not putting yourself above other people		
Calling people names		
Putting other people first by helping them		
Being aggressive and wanting to fight		
Refusing to talk about important issues		
Comforting or caring for people who are sick or old		
Agreeing to do something and then not doing it		
Listening to different points of view		
Being selfish and trying to get the best for yourself		
Accepting that there can be more than one correct answer or more than one way of doing something—not just your way		

16 Which of the following are most likely to influence our behaviour?

A. Our parents and our values
B. Our religious beliefs
C. Other groups on the community
D. How rich and powerful we are

(a) A only
(b) A and B only
(c) A, B and C only
(d) A, B, C and D

17 Which of the following are most likely to be reasons for choosing the food that we eat?

A. The cost and availability of the food
B. The time taken to prepare the food
C. The availability of a safe water supply
D. The food needs of different age groups, like young children, pregnant women or old people

(a) A, B and D only
(b) A, C and D only
(c) B, C and D only
(d) A, B, C and D

18 Answer true or false to the following statements:

a Eating enough of the right kind of food each day is called eating a balanced diet.
b When we eat too much of some types of food, we can become overweight.
c People who are very overweight are called obese.
d Being overweight is healthy but being obese is not healthy.

19 Which of the following statements about food are *true*?

A. Food and drinks that contain a lot of sugar help to make healthy teeth.
B. Food that contains a lot of animal fat or grease can eventually make it hard for blood to move around the body.
C. Foods that contain a lot of salt can cause high blood pressure.

(a) A only
(b) A and B only
(c) B and C only
(d) A, B and C

20 In the tables below, match the use or purpose of food with type of food.

	Use or purpose of food
A	Needed for energy
B	Needed for growth
C	Insulate the body from cold
D	Help the body to work properly
E	Protect the body against sickness
F	Needed to help move waste though the intestines

	Type of food
I	Vitamins
II	Fibre
II	Proteins
IV	Minerals
V	Carbohydrates like starch and sugar
VI	Fats

21 Answer true or false to the following statements.

a Children who are still growing need to eat plenty of protein food.
b Women who are pregnant need to eat less protein and foods like milk that contain calcium, which can harm the baby.
c People who are very active, do hard physical work or play sport need to eat more energy food.
d People who are sick need to eat more food to help them get better.
e People living in a hot place need to eat more energy food than people living in a cold place.
f People living in hot places need to drink plenty of liquids.

22 Which of the following are most likely to be health goals?

A. Take regular exercise and take part in leisure activities
B. Refuse to take drugs
C. Be careless about hygiene and the way that you live

(a) A and B only
(b) A and C only
(c) B and C only
(d) A, B and C

23 Which of the following is *least* likely to be a health goal?

A. Develop positive self-esteem—feel good about yourself and the things that you can do
B. Look for dangerous situations
C. Have good relationships with other people
D. Learn how to deal with difficult and dangerous situations

24 Which of the following are ways to protect yourself and others from harm and stay healthy? Answer true or false.

a Smoke cigarettes with your friends because you want to feel part of the group.
b When you are old enough to drink alcohol, drink only a little.
c Ignore the warning on the bottle about drinking methylated spirits.
d Say 'no' to drugs like marijuana.
e Keep dangerous objects and substances like kerosene and medicines away from children.
f Follow the rules when doing any activity that can be dangerous.
g Go to places where it is unsafe.
h Follow instructions on medicines and bottles of cleaning materials, and other signs.
i Follow directions and given by people in authority like parents, teachers and the police.

25 In the two tables below, match the cause of behaviour with the most likely effect.

	Cause of behaviour
A	Drinking in public places
B	Drinking and driving
C	Chewing and spitting betel nut
D	Throwing rubbish such as bottles
E	Rape
F	Smoking inside buildings

	Effect of behaviour
I	People cutting their feet
II	Sexually transmitted infections
III	People having breathing problems
IV	Road traffic accidents
V	Fighting and damage to property
VI	Stains on buildings and buses

Questions 26–27 refer to the following information on health promotion—the things that we do in order to prevent or reduce sickness and to stay healthy.

A. Health education—teaching people to find out about the causes of sickness and how to stay healthy
B. Immunisation—giving injections or vaccinations
C. Drinking clean water
D. Using toilets properly and keeping them clean
E. Getting rid of rubbish to prevent flies and rats
F. Eating a balanced diet

26 Which of the six steps of health promotion (A–F) can people most easily follow without needing help from other people?
(a) A and B only
(b) A, B, C and D only
(c) C, D, E and F only
(d) A, B, C, D, E and F

27 In which of the six steps of health promotion (A–F) will people most likely need the help of others?
(a) A and B
(b) B and C
(c) C and D
(d) D and E
(e) E and F

28 Which of the following results of development are likely to also have an effect on our health? Answer true or false.
a Polluted rivers and creeks that are used for drinking and fishing
b Cutting down trees that are used for traditional medicine
c Being able to travel from place to place more quickly
d Poisonous chemicals that are used in some mines and plantations

29 In the following list, put a tick in the appropriate column to show which are positive and which are negative effects of producing, selling or using drugs.

Effect of producing, selling or using drugs	Positive effect	Negative effect
Smoking can lead to diseases like lung disease and liver disease		
Farmers earn money from growing and selling tobacco		
Drinking can cause accidents (such as road accidents) and death		
Provincial governments earn money from the tax on beer		
Violence and abuse—especially after getting drunk		
Family breakdown		
Crime—stealing to find money to pay for drugs		
National government earns money from the tax on tobacco		

30 Which of the following are ways that are most likely to help you to say 'no' to the use of drugs?

A. Choose your friends carefully—some people who take drugs may want you to take them too, or you may feel like following them.
B. Learn to make up your own mind and follow your own thinking.
C. Don't follow other people when they are doing something that is illegal or harmful.
C. When people are doing something that is against the law or that is harmful, do not stay with them. Go somewhere else.

(a) A only
(b) A and B only
(c) A, B and C only
(d) A, B, C and D

Chapter 5: Living and Working Together

1 If there is a service organisation nearby, like a Rotary Club or Apex Club, invite someone to come to the school to talk about his or her community service in the area.
2 Invite someone from the community to come and talk about the value of different rules and laws.
3 Invite a policeman or policewoman to come and talk about his or her work in the community.
4 If your school is near a town, find out when the District Court or National Court is sitting and arrange a visit to the court. Or invite a magistrate to visit your school and talk about the work of the courts.
5 Use a questionnaire like the one below to carry out a survey about the attitudes of students in your school and people in the local community. Some questions have been included but you can write more of your own.

	Strongly agree	Agree	Disagree	Strongly disagree
All of the laws in PNG are good laws				
There should be different laws for different people				
Too many leaders in PNG do not follow the Leadership Code				
Leaders who break the law should be punished				

6 Using the words in the list, find the words that are missing from the passages below. You can use each word only once.

ourselves	rights	active	positive	choose	live
freedom	community	leader	choices	roles	

When we take an ____________________ part in the community in which we live, then we help everyone else in the ____________________. There are many things that we can ____________________ to do in the community in order to help others. When we make choices, there can be both ____________________ and negative results which come from those ____________________ . Some choices may affect only ____________________ and other choices will affect other people in the community.

Leaders in the community have particular ____________________ and responsibilities, and the community has expectations about the way that a ____________________ carries out his or her role. Rules and laws are needed to give people the right and ____________________ to live safely and be protected against other people. If ____________________ and freedoms are taken away, then people will be afraid and will not be able to ____________________ safely together.

7 Answer true or false to the following statements about the values that we use to make decisions.

- **a** We can do whatever we like with things that belong to the community.
- **b** We should know and admit when other people are dishonest.
- **c** We should be open-minded and ready to listen.
- **d** We should be quick to judge other people when they do something wrong.
- **e** We should be kind and considerate and understand the feelings of other people.
- **f** We should be cooperative and accept that people are different.
- **g** We should always expect other people to follow our way of doing things.
- **h** We should understand what is happening in the community and take part in community activities.
- **i** We should always think about helping ourselves before we help the community.
- **j** We should treat people equally and respect the rights of other people.
- **k** We can ignore the law if we think there is a better way to sort out a problem.

8 Which of the following are choices that you can make for yourself?

A. How tall you will be
B. To eat properly and exercise regularly
C. Whether to smoke, drink alcohol and take drugs
D. What you will do when you leave school

(a) B and C only
(b) A, B and C only
(c) A, B and D only
(d) B, C and D only

9 Which of the following are examples of choices that are most likely to be important to the community?

A. Taking a position of leadership in the community
B. Deciding whether to get married
C. Helping to solve conflicts between different groups of people
D. Selling cigarettes, alcohol or other drugs

(a) A, B and C
(b) A, B and D
(c) A, C and D
(d) B, C and D

10 Which of the following best describes the most likely order of decisions you will make in your life?

A. When to get married, what to study at school, what to eat and drink
B. Whether to drink alcohol, who to talk to at school, what to do when you leave school
C. Whether to take drugs, whether to drink alcohol, whether to smoke
D. What classmates to make friends with, what to do when you leave school, when to get married

11 Which of the following are things that good leaders should do? Answer true or false.
- **a** Be responsible and ready to answer for the way that they behave
- **b** Help the people who are closest to them, like family and friends
- **c** Be open and honest in dealing with other people
- **d** Behave in ways to show that they are better than other people
- **e** Communicate openly with the community
- **f** Understand the needs and rights of everyone in the community
- **g** Listen to the community and to what other leaders say
- **h** Be prepared to make decisions that most people in the community do not support

12 Which of the following are reasons for having laws? Answer true or false.
- **a** For safety and protection
- **b** To be fair to everyone in the community, so that everyone is treated the same
- **c** To protect criminals from being punished
- **d** To help people to respect public property like schools, churches and playing fields
- **e** To help people to live and work in peace
- **f** To allow mining and logging companies to take resources from the environment

13 Which of the following are values on which rules and laws are based?
- A. Helping people to live a healthy way of life
- B. Encouraging people to share and help each other
- C. Helping people to live as a community and to work together
- D. Developing a feeling of safety in the community
- E. Helping to weaken customs and traditions

- (a) A, B, C and D
- (b) A, B, C and E
- (c) A, B, D and E
- (d) A, C, D and E

14 When people are selfish and think only of themselves, which of the following are likely to happen? Answer true or false.
- **a** Lack of respect for individuals
- **b** Breakdown of law and order in the community
- **c** Bribery and corruption—people being greedy, dishonest and helping themselves
- **d** Fear of violence and fighting in the community

15 When we think about the rights and freedoms of others, which of the following are likely to happen?
- A. Laws will be followed and respected
- B. People will live and behave peacefully
- C. People will not be able find solutions to problems
- D. Conflict can be resolved or settled
- E. Different points of view will be respected

Additional Projects and Investigations

GRADE 8

Chapter 6: Relationships

1 Find out about equality in Papua New Guinea in places where men and women work. When they do the same work, do they earn the same money? Talk to people who are working or to employers, or find out from job advertisements in newspapers.

2 Invite someone from your community who is a role model to come and give a talk at your school. Ask them how they came to be in their position. Did they have role models? In their behaviour, are they always aware that other people may be watching them?

3 Carry out a survey in your community to find out what standards of behaviour are important.

4 Carry out a survey in your community to find out what people think are the characteristics of a good friendship.

5 Social indicators help to tell us about equality and inequality in a community. We can use social indicators to compare communities and populations. Six social indicators for six countries are shown in the graphs on page 172. For each graph, describe the position of Papua New Guinea for that social indicator in relation to the other countries.

Selected Social Indicators

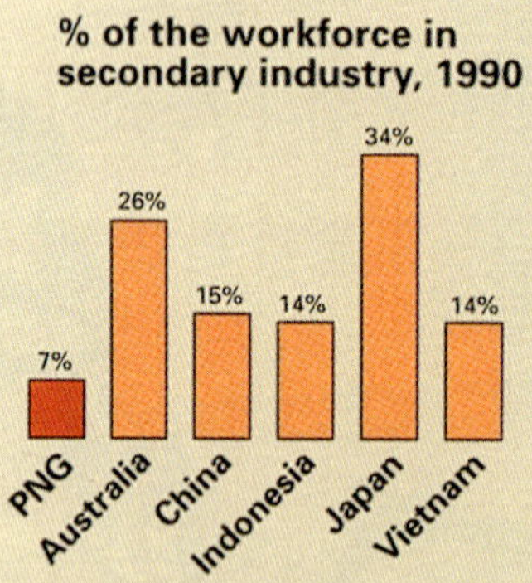

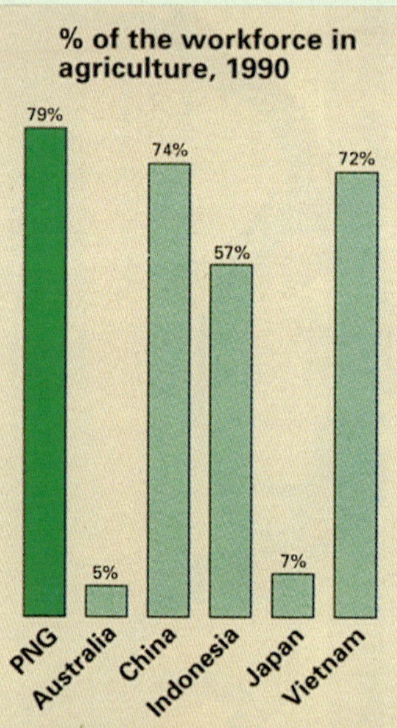

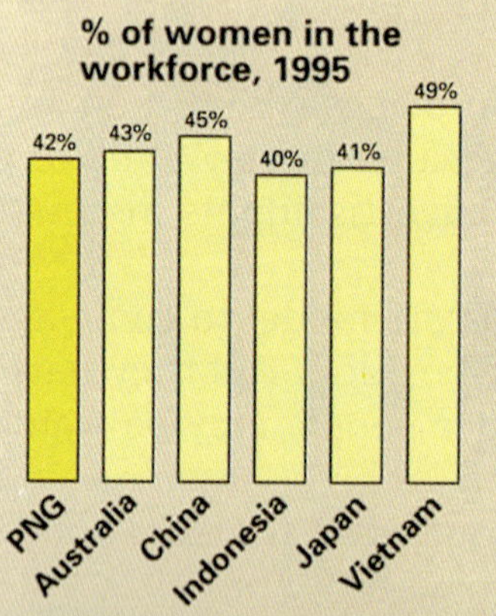

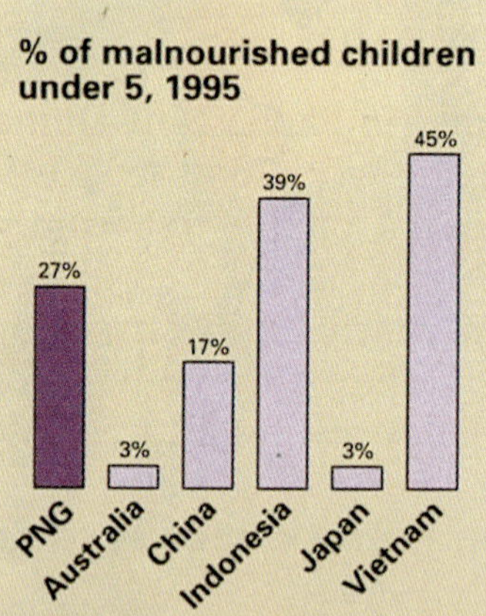

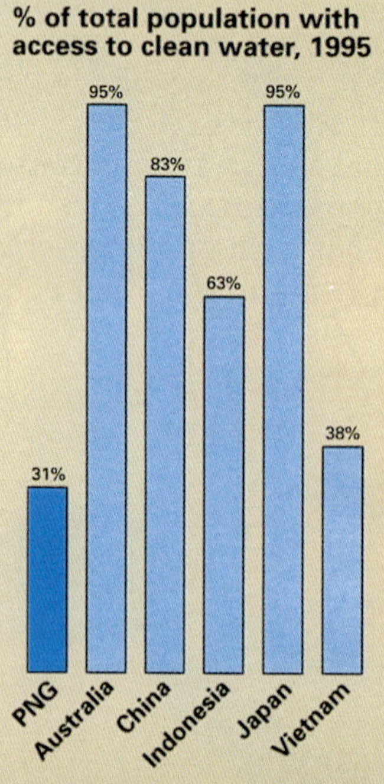

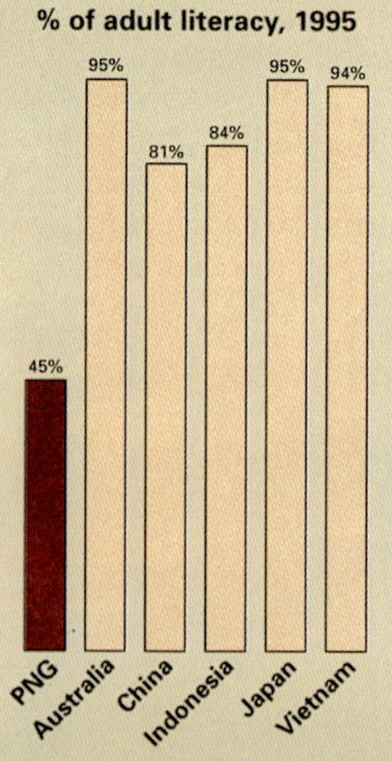

Chapter 7: Movement and Physical Activity

1 Choose a game that is played in your area and play the game, looking for the strategies and tactics that the players use when playing the game. Develop a checklist that you can use to help make and record your observations easily after the game. What conclusions can you make from your observations?

2 Develop a personal fitness program for a number of different people. For example:
A younger brother or sister
An older brother or sister
Your parents
Elderly people
People who are very inactive
People with a disability

3 Choose a game that is played in your area and play the game, looking for the risks that the players take and the rules and safety procedures that are followed in order to reduce the risk. Develop a checklist that you can use to help make and record your observations easily after the game.
- What conclusions can you make from your observations?
- How can the game be made safer?

4 Carry out a survey of any leisure or recreation facilities in your area. Develop a simple form to find the answer to questions such as:
- Who uses the facilities?
- When are they available?
- Are the facilities safe to use?
- Is the equipment that is needed for the activity complete and in working order?
- etc.

Write up a report to summarise your findings.

5 Choose a game that is played in your area and play the game, looking for the ways that the team communicates and cooperates. Develop a checklist that you can use to help make and record your observations easily after the game. What conclusions can you make from your observations?

6 Choose a game that you and your friends like to play. Work out a system of signs or words to communicate with your team-mates about particular moves in the game so that members of the other team will not easily understand. Draw a table with symbols and a key to explain to your team-mates how the system will work.

Example: Basketball
Move 1:
- Player with the ball calls out 'eight'.
- Player with the ball passes it behind the player from the other side who then passes it back to the first player.

Example: Touch
Move 1: The acting-half pass
Watch the ball. Place both hands on the ball and gently swing it from the ground to the receiver. Signal to the team by putting the left foot forward for a pass to the right and the right foot forward for a pass to the left.

Chapter 8: Our Culture, Lifestyle and Values

1 Choose your own community or a community that you know well. Work out a time line to show the customs associated with the seasons, with planting and harvesting of food crops or with other important occasions in the community such as weddings and funerals.

2 Write a letter to invite elders from the community to come and talk about the way that the lifestyle of the people in the area has changed. Show the letter to your teacher before you send it.

3 Invite someone who has lived overseas to come and talk about the way of life of the people in the place where they lived.

4 Invite visitors or people from other places to come and visit your school and talk about their lifestyle. For example, if you live in a place where there are tourists or people travelling on a yacht, you could invite them to come and talk to the students in your school.

Chapter 9: Health of Individuals and Population

1 Plan and cook a nutritious meal for a special occasion and invite some parents from the community to come and share the meal. Or invite some mothers from the community to cook a nutritious meal for your class.

2 Plan a nutrition day for your school. Advertise the day by making posters to put up in the community or by making announcements. Activities could include displays of different kinds of foods, cooking demonstrations, nutritious food to buy and eat, recipes, and stories or poems about food.

3 Invite someone from the local health centre or from the local community to come and give a demonstration on how to plan and prepare nutritious meals using only foods that are available in the local area.

4 Think about the way that people live in your community. Plan and carry out a program to help people to follow healthy practices and live more safely in the community.

First aid for cuts, grazes and scratches

1. Wash with soap and water to remove dirt and microbes.
2. Treat with antiseptic dressing such as gentian violet or Savlon, to kill or stop the growth of bacteria.
3. Cover cleaned area with a bandage or Band-Aid to prevent microbes from entering the wound or flies from sitting on the wound.

Treat symptoms immediately. If the symptoms do not go away, go to the aid-post or clinic.

Keeping people alive

There are a few things that will kill a person in a short time. If you know what to do, you may be able to keep the person alive until you can get help from a health worker.

1. **Stopped breathing.** Check to see if the person has stopped breathing. If a person has stopped breathing, make sure the mouth is clear of any rubbish and give mouth-to-mouth resuscitation. Continue until they are able to breathe by themselves.

2. **Rapid loss of blood.** If a person is losing blood rapidly, you must cover the wound with a piece of cloth or clothing. If nothing else is available, you may have to use your hand to hold the wound closed. Low blood pressure can lead to shock, which is not the same as having a fright.

3. **Stopped heart and circulation.** Check the pulse at the neck or the wrist. If the heart of the person has stopped, you can start the heart again by pushing on the chest and repeating a number of times until the heart beats by itself. However, you must not push too hard, especially with children, so it is best to attend a training course to learn how to do it properly.

4. **Do not leave an unconscious person lying on their back.** When the person is breathing and serious bleeding has been stopped, then you should carefully turn the person on their side so that the tongue, saliva, vomit or blood do not block the airway. This is called the recovery position.

In all these cases you should get help from a health worker as soon as possible.

5 If you find an important health concern that you believe affects many people in your community, discuss this with your teacher. The head teacher of your school, with the Board of Management, may then want to ask the local health inspector to look at the matter.

6 Invite an older person from the community to come and discuss family life in the past and compare it with the present. How many children were in a family then? How was life different?

7 Look at the maps of PNG on pages 176–7 which give information about four health issues in 1994.

- From the information given, which provinces have the best health services? Give reasons for your choice.
- From the information given, which provinces are likely to have the greatest health problems? Give reasons for your choice.

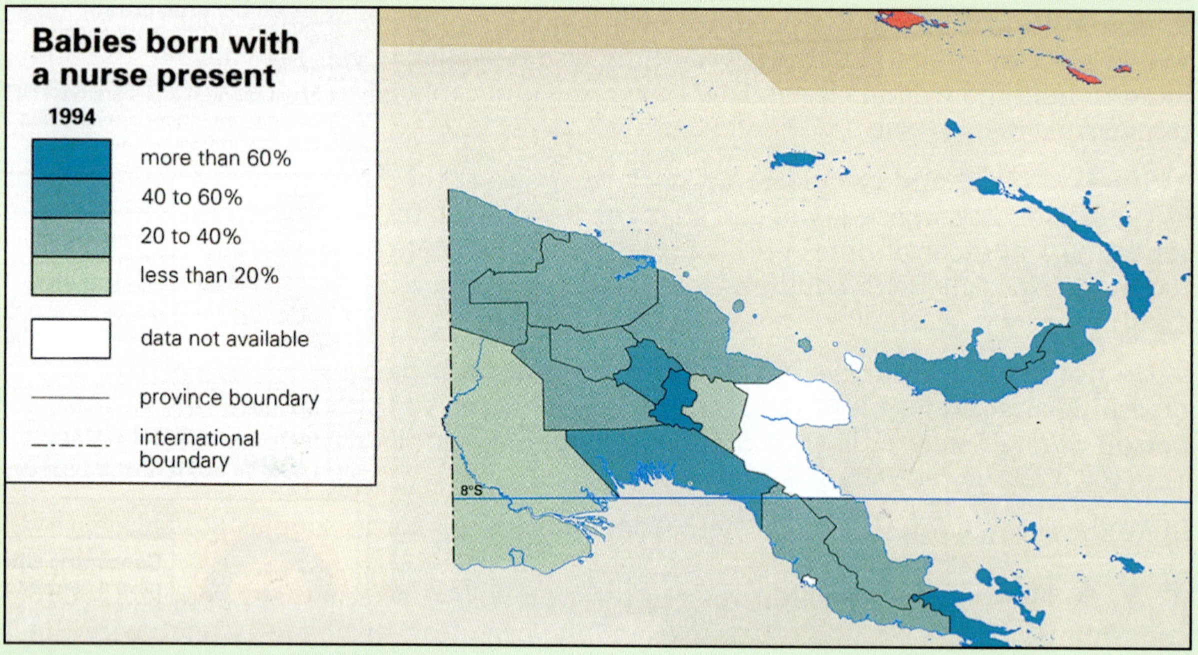
Babies born with a nurse present
1994
more than 60%
40 to 60%
20 to 40%
less than 20%
data not available
province boundary
international boundary
8°S

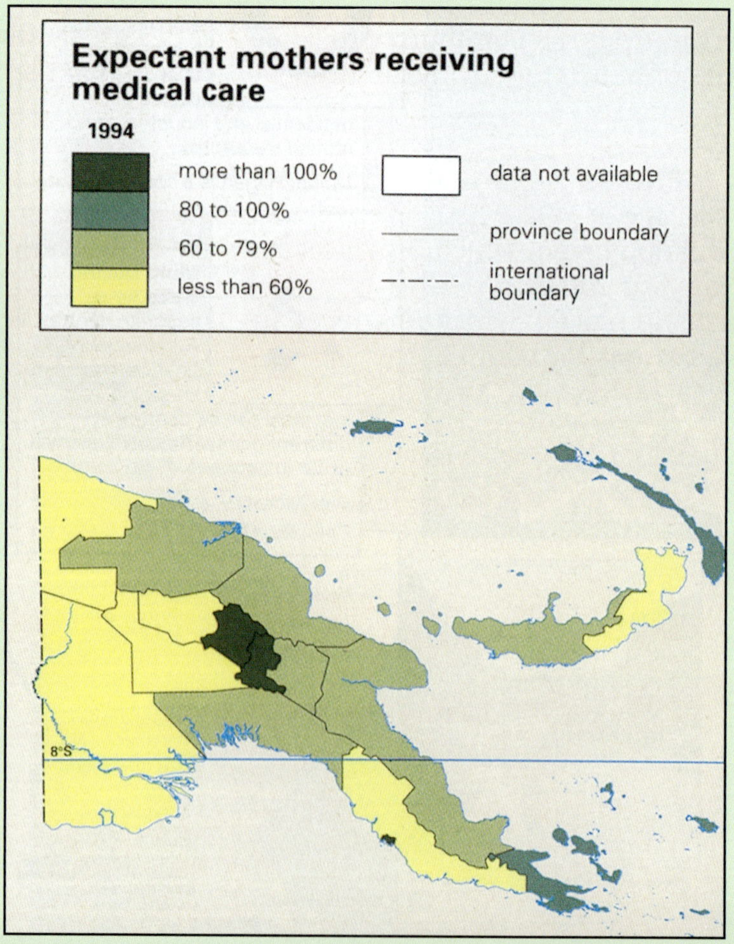
Expectant mothers receiving medical care
1994
more than 100%
80 to 100%
60 to 79%
less than 60%
data not available
province boundary
international boundary
8°S

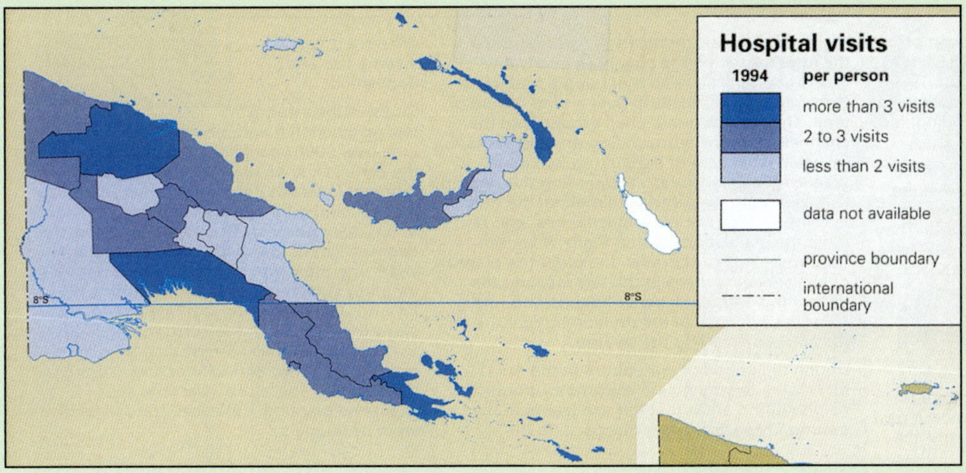

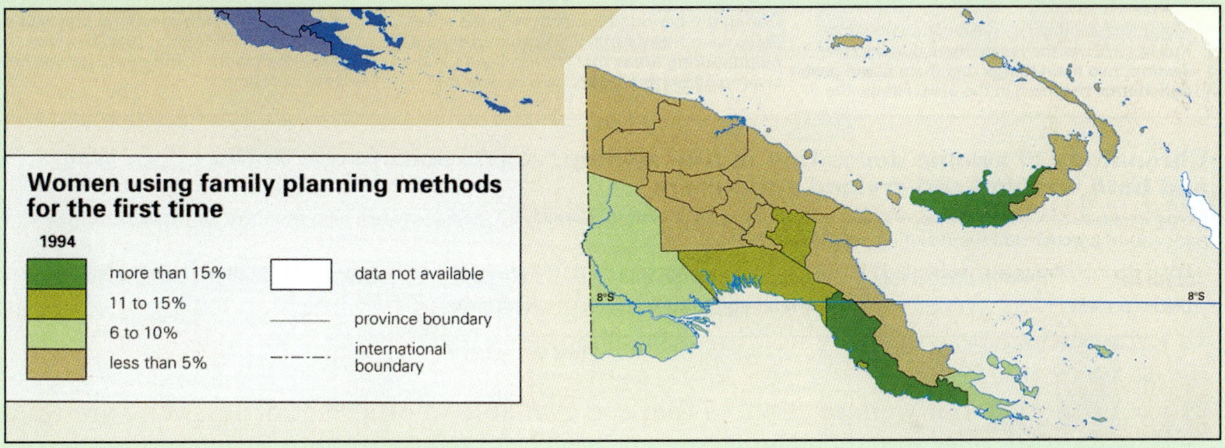

8 Look at the graphs showing cases of diseases preventable by immunisation (1990–93) and total vaccinations (1990–94).

- From the graphs, what are the most important preventable diseases?
- From the graphs, which vaccination program reaches the most children?
- For measles, compare the total vaccinations given with the cases of the disease. What conclusions can you make?

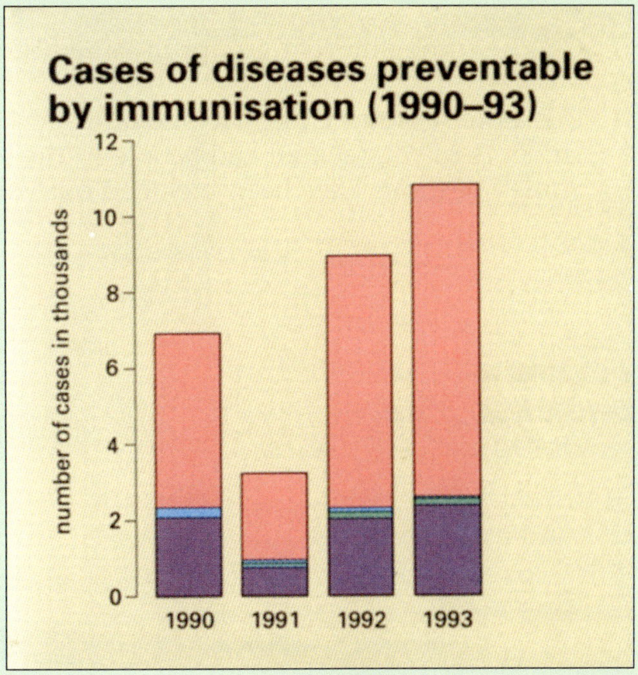

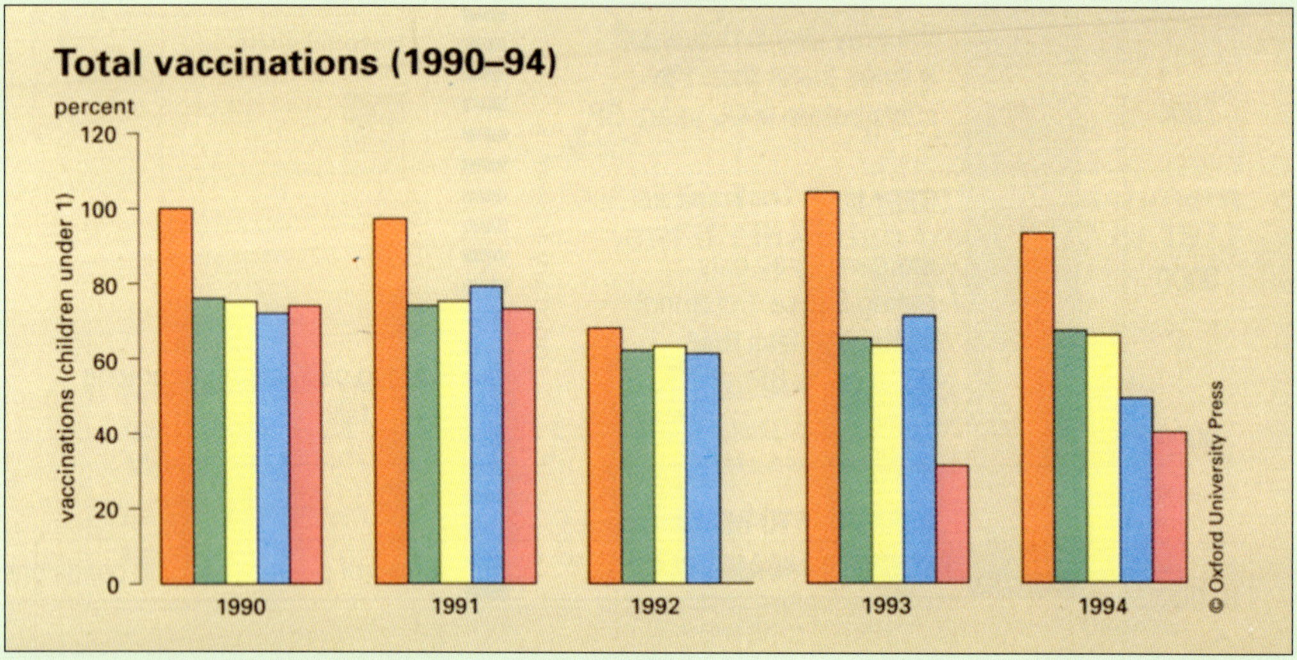

Chapter 10: Living and Working Together

1 Invite a provincial or national politician to come to your school and talk about the way that politicians are elected. You could invite someone who has held a position in the past or someone who is currently holding a position.

2 Find out more about welfare services that are available in other countries. Why are there few welfare services in Papua New Guinea? What can we do to help provide these services?

3 Choose some different groups in Papua New Guinea and find out more about their rights.

4 Use a questionnaire like the one on page 179 to carry out a survey about the ideas of students in your school and people in the local community on rights and responsibilities. Some questions have been included but you can write more of your own.

	Strongly agree	Agree	Disagree	Strongly disagree
Everyone in PNG has freedom of expression and speech to say what they please				
Everyone has equal rights to vote for the best leaders in PNG				
Voting for political leaders should be compulsory				
There is no discrimination in PNG				
Everyone in PNG can live any lifestyle that they choose				
Everyone has equal chance for education in PNG				
Everyone has equal access to health services in both rural and urban areas				

The Community Game

Everyone's a winner!

To play the game you will need

One dice (you can make your own if you do not have one)
One different marker for each player

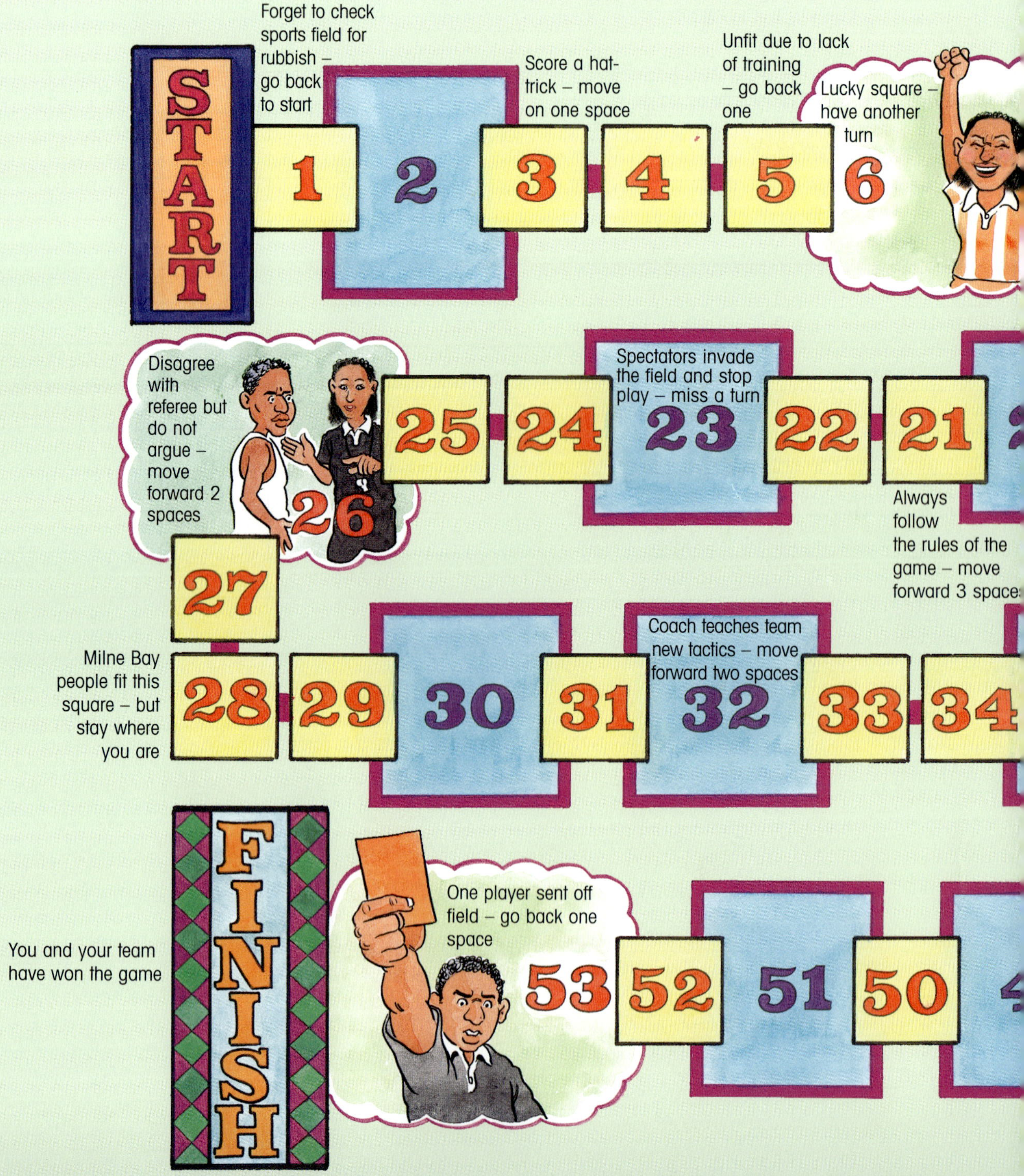

How to play

The first player throws the dice. The number on the dice is the number of squares that the player moves.
Each player then takes a turn.
If you land on a square with writing you must follow the instruction.
The winners are the ones who find themselves in a safe and healthy home.

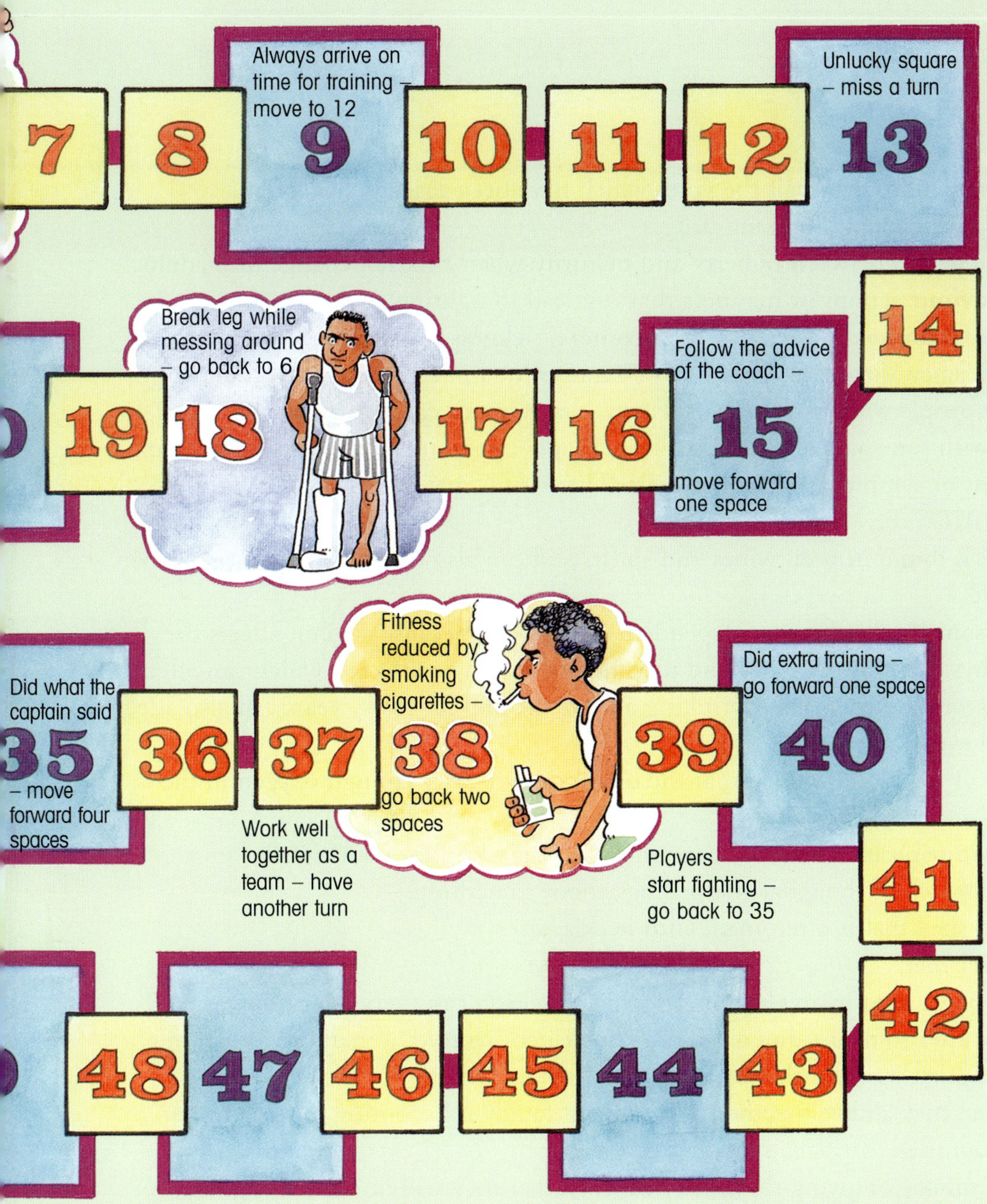
7
8
Always arrive on time for training – move to 12
9
10
11
12
Unlucky square – miss a turn
13
14
Follow the advice of the coach –
15
move forward one space
16
17
Break leg while messing around – go back to 6
18
19
Did what the captain said
35
– move forward four spaces
36
37
Work well together as a team – have another turn
Fitness reduced by smoking cigarettes –
38
go back two spaces
39
Players start fighting – go back to 35
Did extra training – go forward one space
40
41
42
43
44
45
46
47
48

Glossary

absolute majority more than half the votes which have been cast in an election.

addiction being dependent on taking drugs.

adolescence the period between puberty and maturity when children change into adults.

aggressive behaviour actions or manners that can lead to fighting.

AIDS (Acquired Immune Deficiency Syndrome) a sickness caused by the Human Immunodeficiency Virus (HIV) that can be transmitted in semen, vaginal fluid and blood. Most people who catch HIV in Papua New Guinea catch it by having sexual intercourse with someone who has the virus. People can be infected with the virus and show no signs or symptoms for many years. There is no cure for AIDS and most people with AIDS die.

alcohol alcohol is found in beer, wines and spirits and can also be used as an antiseptic or a preservative.

alcoholic a person who has become dependent on alcohol. Because alcohol affects the brain, the physical skills, memory and judgment will also be affected which can affect relationships with other people. Drinking a lot of alcohol for many years can also affect the liver and even cause death.

anaemia a lack of red blood cells so that the blood cannot carry enough oxygen in the body.

assertive behaviour positive behaviour in which you stand up for your rights.

attitude our approach or thoughts and feelings about something.

bagi a small red shell that is often made into necklaces.

balanced diet see diet.

ballot paper a paper used in an election on which a person can mark his or her vote.

blended family after someone dies or after a couple get divorced, a man or woman might get married again. When both husband and wife have children from the previous marriage, then they all live together. This type of family is becoming more common in developed countries.

bribery paying money or giving things to people so that they will do something for you.

candidate a person who stands for election and people can vote for.
carbohydrate a type of food such as sugar and starch which provides energy in the diet.
characteristics qualities that are typical of a person or some other living thing or object.
coach someone who teaches or trains others, for example, in sport.
code of behaviour the ways that we are expected to behave with different people.
components the smaller parts of something that together make the whole.
conception the start of pregnancy when a sperm fertilises an egg in the Fallopian tube. See fertilisation.
concern being kind and interested in other people.
conflict the problems or disagreements that we have with other people.
constipation when people find it difficult or painful to go to the toilet, or when they have hard faeces, then we say they have constipation or are constipated.
contraception a method of preventing pregnancy.
corruption see bribery.
customs the traditions or way of life of people.
de facto a man and woman living together, although they are not married. There may be children in this family, or the couple may not have children.
dedication being keen and loyal and willing to work hard.
dependence (drug dependence) the effect produced when taking a drug becomes a habit. This may include alcohol and 'hard' drugs like heroin and cocaine as well as 'soft' drugs such as tobacco and marijuana.
development 1 the changes that take place in people as they grow from children into adults. **2** the changes that take place in a country.
diabetes a disease in which the person cannot use sugars properly to produce energy. Sugar appears in the urine and the person is thirsty.
diet 1 the mixture of foods that people eat. It is important to eat the right amount of food from the three food groups, which are growth foods such as protein, energy foods such as carbohydrates and protective foods such as fresh fruit and vegetables. This is called a balanced diet. **2** to control the type and amount of food that you eat.
digestive system the system of the body that breaks down food, beginning with the mouth and ending with the anus.
discrimination treating people differently or unfairly because of the place they are from or because of their gender, or because they are disabled.
duties the jobs or activities that people have to do or responsibilities that they must carry out.
economic the way that people earn and use money.
ejaculation the process in which semen is forced out of the penis. This usually happens during sexual intercourse.
election campaign the activities that supporters do in order to help a person to win an election.
environment the surroundings which may influence our growth, development and behaviour. See physical, economic and social.

equality being fair, having the same rights as each other and the same amount of power in a relationship.

expectations the things that we should do or the ways that we should behave.

extended family a family consisting of children, their parents, grandparents and possibly uncles and aunts living closely together.

Fallopian tube (oviduct) the tube that carries eggs from the ovary to the uterus.

family planning deciding on the number of children that a couple want to have and the spacing between the births of those children. Contraception can be used in family planning.

fat one of three types of food that is needed in the diet.

fertilisation the joining together of a sperm and an egg cell. See conception.

fibre (roughage) the part of food that cannot be digested and absorbed to produce energy. Highly refined foods such as white rice, white sugar and white flour contain little fibre. Foods such as fruit and vegetables, nuts and brown rice contain a lot of fibre. People who have a lot of fibre in their diet do not usually have health problems such as constipation, being overweight or diabetes.

first past the post a way of deciding the winner in an election—the person who gets more votes than anybody else.

food chain the way in which some animals eat plants and some animals eat other animals, so that food is passed from one to another.

freedoms the choices that everyone should be allowed to make.

gender being male or female.

germs small living things that can make us sick.

gut feeling the feeling that we get inside our bodies that tells us that something is all right or is not all right.

haus tambaran a traditional house. The front of Parliament Haus in Port Moresby is built in the shape of a Sepik haus tambaran.

hazard a danger that is found in our surroundings.

health goals things that we try to achieve in order to be fit and well.

health promotion all the things that we do to prevent or reduce sickness.

HIV (human immunodeficiency virus) the virus that affects the immune system of the body and leads to **AIDS**.

identity individuality or personality.

immunisation a way of preventing sickness by giving a person an injection or vaccination. Most immunisations are given to children so parents must take their children to the clinic to get them immunised.

inequality something that is not fair or equal.

infant a child under one year of age. A child that cannot live without its mother.

inherited obtained from our parents.

injection forcing drugs or some other liquid into a part of the body by using a syringe.

instinct a skill or behaviour that people have without knowing or being able to explain why.

justice being fair and treating people equally.

kula a trading relationship amongst people in the islands of Milne Bay Province in which shell necklaces are passed in one direction in a circle and armlets are passed in the opposite direction.

Leadership Code a set of rules for Members of Parliament and Senior Public Servants to follow.

leisure free time.

level of intimacy the closeness that people feel in a relationship.

lifestyle the way that people choose to live their lives, which varies from place to place and from time to time.

Limited Preferential Voting (LPV) a system of electing a person in which the candidate must receive an absolute majority, or more than half the votes counted, in order to win.

linesman someone who helps the referee or umpire to decide if the ball has crossed the line in a game of sport.

locomotor skills the skills that we use when we move from place to place, like running, swimming.

malnutrition not eating the amount and type of food that is needed to be healthy. This is very important when children are still growing.

menstruation see period.

microbe any living thing that is too small to be seen with the naked eye; for example bacteria, viruses and some fungi and protozoa.

mineral a substance found in food in small amounts that is important for good health.

modern societies people living a way of life which is typical for the present time and continues to change with the times.

nicotine the drug found in tobacco and which is addictive. See addiction.

nominations choosing a person as a candidate in an election.

non-locomotor skills the skills that we use when we move but stay in the same place, like hitting a ball.

nourishing food that is healthy and satisfying.

nuclear family a family consisting of children and their parents living together.

nutrients the substances found in food which give energy and help us to grow and stay healthy.

nutrition 1 the food that people eat and the way that their bodies use that food. **2** the study of food.

obesity people who are very overweight are obese.

obligations the things that we are expected to do.

Ombudsman Commission an organisation set up by the government to deal with complaints against leaders. See also Leadership Code.

overweight being heavier than average for your height and age.

passive smoking breathing in the smoke which comes from the tobacco that other people are smoking.

peer pressure feeling that you have to behave in a particular way because other people of your age behave in that way.

period when a girl or woman has a period, a small amount of blood and mucus flows from the uterus out of the vagina. Periods start when a girl is about 13 and continue about once a month until the age of 45–55, when they stop. This is a perfectly natural thing to happen and a woman having her period is not dirty and can do normal things. When a girl starts to have her periods it means that she can have a baby and when she is pregnant her periods stop; missing a period is often the first sign that a woman is pregnant.

physical the appearance or surroundings.

pollution waste produced by the activities of people that can affect the land, rivers, the sea and air.

polyandry when a woman has more than one husband. The woman may have children who have different fathers. Polyandry is one kind of polygamy.

polygamy when a man has more than one wife, or a woman has more than one husband, this is called polygamy. Polygamy is found in some parts of Papua New Guinea.

polygyny when a man has more than one wife. The man may have children with each of his wives. Each wife may live in her own house away from the other wives to prevent arguments. Polygyny is one kind of polygamy.

protein a type of food in the diet that, after being digested, is used in growth to form muscles, tissues and organs. Also known as growth food.

puberty the period of sexual development.

pubic area the area around the penis or vagina.

recreation things that we do to relax and enjoy ourselves. See leisure.

referee a person who controls a game of sport.

respect the way that we treat ourselves and others, laws and property.

responsibility being trustworthy and able to answer for the way that you behave. The job that a person has to do.

rights the things that people are allowed to have or do because of the law or because it is correct.

risk a behaviour that can have a bad effect on our health or well-being.

role the part that a person plays in a family, at school, in a sports team etc.

safety procedures things that we can do to deal with danger and keep ourselves safe.

scrotum the bag of skin that holds the testicles. The scrotum helps to keep the testicles at a lower temperature than the rest of the body, which is better for producing and storing sperm.

semen the creamy liquid that contains sperm and that comes out of the penis during ejaculation.

sex 1 being a male or a female. **2** sexual contact between a man and a woman.

sexual development the changes that take place in our bodies as we develop from a girl to a woman and a boy into a man. See also puberty.

sexuality the way that we think, feel and behave because we are a male or a female.

sexually transmitted disease (STD) another term for sexually transmitted infection.

sexually transmitted infection (STI) (venereal disease) any disease which can be transmitted during sexual intercourse. Most STIs are caused by bacteria and can be cured by antibiotics if the person gets treatment early enough. AIDS, Donovanosis, gonorrhoea and syphilis are all STIs.

single parent family a family in which there is only a mother or a father to take care of the children.

spectators people watching a game of sport.

sperm the male sex cell. Sperm are usually found in semen and a single sperm fertilises the egg at the time of conception.

staple food the main food that people eat every day, like sweet potato, yam, banana.

stereotyping forming an opinion or making a judgment about somebody without having good reasons, especially when we think that a person has the characteristics of other members of the group.

strategy a plan to help achieve goals or objectives. See also tactics.

stretching exercises that people do before playing sport which help the muscles and joints.

submissive behaviour being quiet and passive.

subsistence agriculture growing and eating your own food; many people in Papua New Guinea do this.

suburbs the outer areas of a city.

survive to stay alive, to carry on.

symptoms something that a person notices which shows that the person is sick.

tactics the things that people do in order to achieve a particular purpose, like winning a game of sport. See also strategy.

tally room the place where votes are counted in an election.

testicles (balls) the two male sex organs which are held in the scrotum. The testicles produce sperm.

tolerance accepting other people and their behaviour without being critical.

traditional societies people who still follow the customs and rules that were followed by their parents and grandparents.

travel move from place to place, for example, when playing sport.

vaccination a way of protecting a person against a disease. A vaccine is usually given by injection, but can also be given by mouth and scratching the skin. See immunity.

values the things that people say or think are important.

vitamin a substance found in fresh fruit and vegetables in small amounts that is important for good health.

voters the people who are able to vote in an election.

wet dream semen which comes out of a boy's penis when he is asleep.

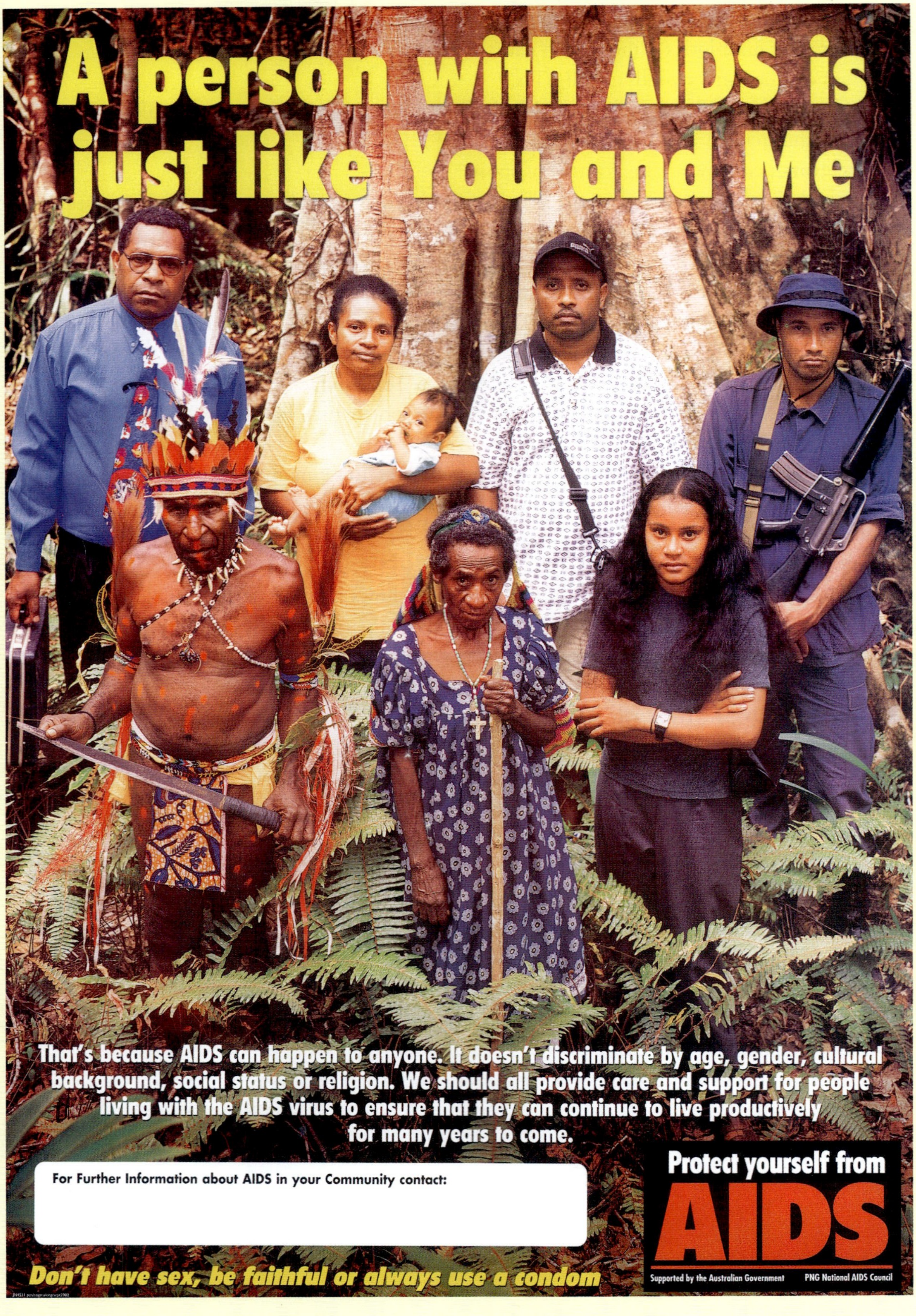
A person with AIDS is just like You and Me
That's because AIDS can happen to anyone. It doesn't discriminate by age, gender, cultural background, social status or religion. We should all provide care and support for people living with the AIDS virus to ensure that they can continue to live productively for many years to come.
For Further Information about AIDS in your Community contact:
Protect yourself from
AIDS
Supported by the Australian Government
PNG National AIDS Council
Don't have sex, be faithful or always use a condom